Design, Develop, Deliver
Using ADDIE to Build Effective Healthcare Simulations

Keith A. Beaulieu

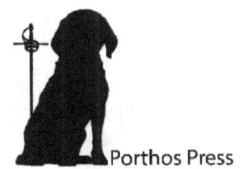

KEITH A. BEAULIEU

**Design, Develop, Deliver
Using ADDIE to Build Effective Healthcare Simulations**

Copyright © 2025 by Keith A. Beaulieu, Porthos Press
All Rights Reserved.

No part of this document may be reproduced or transmitted in any form or by any means, electronic, mechanical, photocopying, recording, or otherwise, without prior written permission.

Requests for permission to make copies of any part of the work should be submitted to the publisher.

Published by Keith A. Beaulieu, Porthos Press
Contact@porthospress.com

Printed in the United States of America
First Printing: 2025

ISBN 978-1-7360792-8-7 (Paperback)

First edition, 2025
10 9 3 7 6 5 4 3 2 1

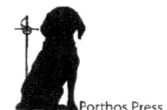

Contents

Introduction 1

Chapter 1 Understanding The Addie Model 7

Chapter 2 Analyze Phase in Healthcare Simulation 21

Chapter 3 Designing the Curriculum 53

Chapter 4 Development 71

Chapter 5 Implementation in Healthcare Simulation 87

Chapter 6 Evaluation and Feedback 103

Chapter 7 Resource Allocation Across Phases in the Addie Model 119

Chapter 8 Linking Addie to Competency Frameworks 131

Chapter 9 Iterative Refinement in the Addie Model 137

Chapter 10 Scaling Simulations Across Learner Levels 145

Chapter 11 Interdisciplinary Applications of the Addie Model 155

Chapter 12 Case Studies 163

Chapter 13 Criticisms of the Addie Model for Healthcare Simulation and Adaptations for Flexibility 171

Chapter 14 Quality Control in Addie – Ensuring Validity and Reliability of Checklists and Rubrics 181

Chapter 15 The Future of Addie in Healthcare Simulation 191

Conclusion 201

Appendices 206

About the Author 269

Analyze
- Needs Assessment
- Resources Needed
- Draft Budget and timeline (as needed)

Design
- Rationale
- Goal and objectives
- Learner Profile/learner prerequisites
- Course/activity description
- Debriefing strategy
- Evaluation strategy
- Plan deliverables

Develop
- Lesson plan
- Scenario development
- Evaluation checklist
- Job Aids
- Pilot test

Implement
- Make active
- Evaluate activity/debrief team (ops team & content experts)
- Modify activity as needed

Evaluate
- Review all ADDIE elements
- Review that all goals and objectives were met
- Provide report to stakeholders
- Surveys

"Develop a passion for learning. If you do, you will never cease to grow."
— Anthony J. D'Angelo

Introduction

Purpose of the Book

Healthcare simulation is invaluable for teaching, learning, and assessing skills in a controlled and safe environment. However, the effectiveness of simulation-based education relies heavily on its design and implementation. Simulations can fail to meet learning objectives without a structured approach, leaving participants inadequately prepared for real-world challenges.

Imagine a scenario where a group of nursing students manages a critically ill patient in a simulated environment. The learning potential is immense—from clinical decision-making to teamwork and communication. However, without a well-thought-out design, the simulation might miss key learning objectives or fail to provide meaningful feedback. This is where the ADDIE model shines. By offering a step-by-step framework, ADDIE ensures that every aspect of the simulation, from its initial goals to its final evaluation, is meticulously planned and executed.

This book aims to bridge that gap by demonstrating how the ADDIE model—a proven framework for instructional design—can be used to create effective, engaging, and impactful healthcare simulations. ADDIE, which stands for Analysis, Design, Development, Implementation, and Evaluation, offers a systematic method to design and deliver educational experiences that are both purposeful and outcome-driven. Educators and instructional designers can use ADDIE to ensure that every simulation is engaging and aligned with clear learning goals and measurable outcomes.

The importance of structured instructional design cannot be overstated in a field where patient safety and clinical competence are critical. This book provides the tools and insights needed to craft simulations that truly prepare healthcare professionals for the complexities of their work. Through the lens of ADDIE, you will discover how to transform a simple idea into a powerful educational experience that leaves a lasting impact.

Target Audience

This book is written for a diverse audience of professionals dedicated to excellence in healthcare education and training. It is designed for:
- **Educators** seeking to enhance their teaching methodologies with evidence-based practices in simulation design.
- **Instructional Designers** tasked with creating comprehensive simulation programs that align with educational and organizational goals.
- **Healthcare Professionals** who utilize simulation to train staff, improve team dynamics, or assess competencies.

Picture an educator standing before a group of eager learners, ready to launch into a simulation designed to teach life-saving skills. Or imagine an instructional designer working behind the scenes, meticulously crafting scenarios that mirror the complexity of real-life medical emergencies. These are the individuals this book seeks to empower. Whether you are new to simulation or an experienced practitioner looking to refine your approach, this guide will provide practical strategies and a deeper understanding of how to apply the ADDIE model effectively in your work.

Overview

The ADDIE model has long been a cornerstone of instructional design across various industries, and its application to healthcare simulation is both logical and highly effective. Think of it as a blueprint—one that guides you from the initial spark of an idea to the polished execution of a fully realized simulation. Imagine embarking on a journey where each step builds upon the last, taking you from identifying the needs of your learners to witnessing the transformative impact of a well-executed simulation.

In this book, you will explore each phase of ADDIE—Analysis, Design, Development, Implementation, and Evaluation—through the lens of healthcare simulation. In the Analysis phase, you'll uncover strategies to dig deep into learner needs and organizational goals. In the Design phase, you will see how to craft scenarios that resonate, capturing the nuances of real-life clinical situations. The Development phase will guide you through the process of turning these plans into tangible tools, from mannequins and software to detailed role-play scripts. When it comes to Implementation, you will discover best practices for delivering simulations that inspire confidence and competence. Finally, the Evaluation phase will equip you with tools to measure success, adapt for improvement, and close the loop on the educational experience.

This journey is not just about process—it is about transformation. Imagine the sense of accomplishment when your carefully designed simulation enables a healthcare team to respond effectively to a critical situation, potentially saving lives. Picture the confidence in your learners as they step into the real world, armed with skills honed through your simulations. Through detailed examples, case studies, and practical tips, this book will show you how the ADDIE model can be your compass, guiding you to create simulations that are as impactful as they are educational.

By the end of this book, you will have a clear roadmap for creating simulations that are pedagogically sound and practical and impactful in real-world healthcare settings. Whether designing a single simulation or building an entire curriculum, this book will serve as your comprehensive guide to success. Let us embark on this journey together, discovering how to design, develop, and deliver simulations that truly make a difference.

A Note about the ADDIE Framework

Although the primary focus of this work is to demonstrate how the ADDIE framework can be utilized to design, develop, and deliver healthcare simulations, it is essential to recognize that ADDIE is a versatile instructional systems design model that extends far beyond simulation. At its core, ADDIE provides a structured and systematic approach to curriculum development that can be applied to a variety of educational contexts. Its iterative and flexible process ensures that learning objectives are clearly defined, instructional strategies are effectively implemented, and outcomes are thoroughly evaluated, making it applicable to virtually any form of training or education.

The ADDIE framework can be adapted to design workshops, didactic lectures, foundational courses, and Objective Structured Clinical Examinations (OSCEs). It is equally useful in creating skills-based training programs and human simulations with standardized patients, where learners can practice communication, assessment, and procedural techniques in a controlled environment. By applying ADDIE's stages—Analyze, Design, Develop, Implement, and Evaluate—educators can ensure that the curriculum is tailored to meet the needs of their learners, whether they are mastering a specific clinical skill or developing critical thinking in a lecture-based setting. This adaptability underscores ADDIE's value as a foundational model for education in both healthcare and beyond.

The True Costs of Curriculum Development and Training

Substantial investments are made annually in curriculum development and training across various sectors in the United States. Educational institutions, employers, and government programs collectively contribute to these expenditures, reflecting a commitment to enhancing skills and competencies nationwide.

Total Expenditures

According to a 2022 report by Credential Engine, total education and training spending in the U.S. was around $2.133 trillion. Educational institutions accounted for about $1.430 trillion, making up roughly

67% of the total expenditure. Employers contributed approximately $594 billion, which equals 28% of the total spending, while state and federal grants, along with military programs, represented the remaining $109 billion, or 5% of the overall expenditures (Credential Engine, 2022).

Per Employee Training Costs
Focusing on employer-sponsored training, data from Statista indicates that the average expenditure on learning and development per employee worldwide has fluctuated over the years. While specific figures for 2022 are unavailable, there was a general trend of increasing investment in employee development leading up to 2019, followed by a slight decline in 2020 and a subsequent increase in 2021 (Statista, n.d.).

Training Hours per Employee
In terms of time investment, employees received an average of 42.1 hours of training per year, according to a 2019 report by *Training Magazine*. This was a slight decrease from 46.7 hours in the previous year. Notably, small companies provided the most hours of training, averaging 49.8 hours per employee annually (*Training Magazine*, 2019).

Educational Institutions' Spending per Student
At the K-12 education level, the National Center for Education Statistics reported that total expenditures for public elementary and secondary schools in the 2020–21 academic year amounted to $927 billion. This translates to an average of $18,614 spent per public school pupil enrolled during that period (National Center for Education Statistics [NCES], n.d.).

These statistics underscore the significant financial resources allocated to curriculum development and training in the United States. The investments span educational institutions, corporate training programs, and government initiatives, highlighting a nationwide commitment to fostering education and professional development.

References

Credential Engine. (2022). *Education and training expenditures in the U.S. (2022 report)*. Retrieved from https://credentialengine.org/resources/education-and-training-expenditures-in-the-u-s-2022-report/

National Center for Education Statistics (NCES). (n.d.). *Public school expenditures*. Retrieved from https://nces.ed.gov/programs/coe/indicator/cmb

Statista. (n.d.). *Average spending on employee training worldwide*. Retrieved from https://www.statista.com/statistics/738519/workplace-training-spending-per-employee/

Training Magazine. (2019). *2019 training industry report*. Retrieved from https://trainingmag.com/2019-training-industry-report/

Chapter 1

Understanding the ADDIE Model

Origins and Evolution

The ADDIE model's origins date back to World War II, when the U.S. military recognized the need for efficient and scalable training methods. During the war, thousands of personnel required rapid training in technical and operational skills, leading to the development of **programmed instruction** and systematic approaches (Reiser & Dempsey, 2017). These methods emphasized breaking complex tasks into smaller, teachable units and aligning instruction with specific objectives.

<u>Early Developments in the 1940s and 1950s</u>

Programmed Instruction: A foundational concept programmed instruction used step-by-step teaching to improve learner retention and reduce training errors. This approach laid the groundwork for the systematic methods later used in ADDIE.

- **Systems Approach**: As training expanded in complexity, the military applied engineering-inspired systems approaches, emphasizing process control, feedback loops, and continuous improvement (Gagné et al., 2005).

Transition to Systematic Design in the 1960s and 1970s

In the 1960s, the demand for instructional systems grew as education and corporate sectors sought scalable solutions for training. Influential theories emerged during this time, such as Robert Gagné's *Nine Events of Instruction*, which provided a structured way to sequence learning and align it with cognitive objectives. Gagné's work influenced ADDIE's design and development phases, particularly its focus on clearly defined outcomes and evidence-based practices (Morrison et al., 2013).

The ADDIE model began to take shape in the early 1970s when Florida State University's Center for Educational Technology developed it for the U.S. Army. It was initially designed to standardize training development through the Instructional Systems Design (ISD) framework, ensuring systematic alignment between training objectives, instructional methods, and evaluation processes (Allen, 2006).

The central principle of ADDIE is systematic thinking. By dividing the instructional design process into distinct yet interconnected phases, ADDIE guarantees that each step builds on the previous one, resulting in a coherent and effective learning experience (Morrison et al., 2013). This iterative approach facilitates ongoing refinement, ensuring that instructional materials are well-designed and responsive to the needs of learners and organizations.

The ADDIE model offers an invaluable framework in healthcare simulation, where precision and realism are essential. Its structured approach aligns seamlessly with the challenges of designing simulations that replicate real-world clinical settings. By utilizing ADDIE, educators and instructional designers can develop purposeful, engaging, and impactful simulations (Branch, 2009).

Widespread Adoption

ADDIE gained popularity across multiple industries after its development for the U.S. Army. By the 1980s, it was a standard corporate training, education, and healthcare framework. The structured phases of ADDIE allowed for systematic training design, ensuring programs met their objectives efficiently. For example, a study by Reigeluth (1999) found that systematic approaches like ADDIE improved learning outcomes by an average of 25% compared to unstructured training methods.

Influences on ADDIE's Development

Several key theories and frameworks influenced the development and refinement of ADDIE:

- **Gagné's Conditions of Learning**
  Gagné's framework emphasized aligning instruction with cognitive processes, such as recall, comprehension, and problem-solving (Gagné et al., 2005). This theory shaped ADDIE's Analysis and Design phases by encouraging instructional designers to consider how learners process information.

- **Bloom's Taxonomy**
  Benjamin Bloom's hierarchical model of learning objectives (cognitive, affective, psychomotor) provided a foundation for creating clear, measurable outcomes within ADDIE (Bloom, 1956). For example, instructional designers could use Bloom's framework to define objectives like "demonstrate proficiency in CPR" or "analyze the causes of patient deterioration."

- **Systems Thinking**
  ADDIE reflects the influence of systems theory, emphasizing interdependence among its phases. For example, insights gained during evaluation often inform refinements in design and development, creating a feedback loop for continuous improvement (Branch, 2009).

Core Elements of the Model

Each phase of the ADDIE model plays a critical role in the instructional design process. Let's delve into the details of each phase:

Analyze The Analysis phase lays the groundwork for the entire project. During this phase, instructional designers identify the needs of the learners, define the learning objectives, and consider the constraints and resources available. Key questions addressed in this phase include:

- Who are the learners, and what are their current knowledge and skills?
- What gaps exist between current competencies and desired outcomes?
- What organizational goals should the instruction support?

In healthcare simulation, the analysis might involve understanding the clinical skills learners need to develop, such as managing cardiac arrests or performing surgical procedures. The insights gained during this phase inform every subsequent step (Gagné et al., 2005).

Design The Design phase translates the insights from Analysis into a concrete plan. This includes defining learning objectives, selecting instructional methods, and outlining the content structure. Design also involves planning for assessment, ensuring that learning outcomes can be measured effectively (Reigeluth, 1999).

For example, in a simulation to train nurses in neonatal resuscitation, the design phase might involve creating a detailed scenario script, specifying the equipment required, and identifying the roles of facilitators and learners.

Develop The Development phase brings the design plan to life. This is where instructional materials, such as simulation scenarios, guides, and assessment tools, are created. Development often involves collaboration among subject matter experts, educators, and technical staff to ensure accuracy and realism (Dick et al., 2005).

For instance, a high-fidelity simulation of a trauma case might require the development of lifelike mannequins, realistic patient monitors, and digital resources for pre-briefing and debriefing.

Implement Implementation is the phase where the simulation is delivered to learners. This involves running the simulation and managing logistical details, such as scheduling, setting up the environment, and preparing facilitators. During this phase, it is crucial to ensure that learners are adequately briefed and that facilitators are equipped to guide the experience (Branch, 2009).

In healthcare simulation, implementation often includes pilot sessions to identify and resolve issues before full deployment.

Evaluate The Evaluation phase assesses the instructional intervention's effectiveness. This includes formative evaluation, conducted during the development and implementation phases, and summative evaluation, conducted after the simulation. Key metrics might include learner performance, satisfaction, and the achievement of learning objectives (Kirkpatrick & Kirkpatrick, 2006).

For example, a simulation designed to improve communication in surgical teams might evaluate success using observation checklists, self-assessments, and patient outcome data.

ADDIE Process

Phase	Purpose	Key Questions	Outputs
Analyze	Identify training needs, target audience, and learning objectives.	- What performance gaps exist? - Who are the learners? - What are the organizational goals this simulation supports?	- **Training Needs**: Example: Improve cardiac arrest management. - **Learner Profile**: Example: Second-year nursing students. - **Learning Objectives**: Example: Demonstrate effective use of ACLS protocols.

Phase	Purpose	Key Questions	Outputs
Design	Create a detailed blueprint for the simulation.	- What specific learning outcomes should the simulation achieve? - What instructional methods will be used? - What assessments will evaluate learner performance?	- **Scenario Outline:** Example: Cardiac arrest scenario requiring teamwork. - **Learning Objectives:** Perform high-quality CPR. - **Assessment Plan:** Checklist for skills and communication.

DESIGN, DEVELOP, DELIVER: USING ADDIE TO BUILD EFFECTIVE HEALTHCARE SIMULATIONS

Phase	Purpose	Key Questions	Outputs
Develop	Build materials and resources based on the design blueprint.	- What tools and resources are needed to implement the simulation? - Are facilitators trained and prepared?	- **Simulation Materials:** Scenario script, mannequin programming, debriefing guides. - **Pre-Briefing Materials:** Handouts on ACLS protocols. - Facilitator **Training:** Orientation for facilitators.

Phase	Purpose	Key Questions	Outputs
Implement	Deliver the simulation to learners and gather initial feedback.	- Are the logistics and environment prepared? - Are facilitators equipped to manage the simulation and debriefing?	- **Execution Plan:** Example: Schedule simulations for groups of six participants. - **Logistics Checklist:** Room setup, equipment check. - **Observation Notes:** Document learner behavior.

Phase	Purpose	Key Questions	Outputs
Evaluate	Assess the simulation's effectiveness and identify areas for improvement.	- Did learners achieve the intended outcomes? - What improvements can be made for future iterations?	- **Formative Evaluation:** Example: Facilitator feedback on pacing. - **Summative Evaluation:** Learner performance data, feedback surveys. - **Recommendations:** Adjust complexity based on skill levels.

ADDIE: Key Concepts

The ADDIE model is built upon foundational principles ensuring systematic, measurable, and learner-centered instruction. These key concepts are the backbone of the model, guiding the development of effective training programs and ensuring that educational goals are met with precision and accountability. Below, we explore the essential concepts that define ADDIE's approach and highlight why it remains a cornerstone in instructional design.

1. **Instruction Is Based on Job Requirements**
   One of the primary tenets of ADDIE is that the instruction content is directly tied to the skills and knowledge required for a specific job or role. In healthcare simulation, this means that training scenarios must reflect the responsibilities and challenges professionals face. For example, a simulation for ICU nurses might focus on managing patient deterioration because this is a critical and frequent part of their role. By grounding instruction in job-specific tasks, ADDIE ensures relevance and practical application.

2. **Objectives Are Derived from Behavioral Analysis**
   The learning objectives in ADDIE are rooted in a detailed analysis of behavior and performance needs. These objectives are crafted to be measurable and observable, ensuring that the success of the instruction can be evaluated effectively. For instance, a simulation on sepsis management might include objectives such as "recognize early signs of septic shock" or "demonstrate proper administration of vasopressors." This focus on observable outcomes allows facilitators to assess whether learners meet the required standards.

3. **Targeted Instruction**
   ADDIE emphasizes that instruction should address only the gaps in knowledge or skills that learners have not yet mastered. This concept ensures efficiency and prevents redundancy. For instance, before a simulation, learners might complete a pre-assessment to identify areas of weakness, and the instruction would then focus solely on those areas. This targeted approach optimizes learning time and maximizes impact.

4. **Criterion-Referenced Measurement**
   Measurement in ADDIE is tied directly to the learning objectives, with learners evaluated against established criteria rather than being compared to their peers. This ensures that

the focus remains on individual performance and mastery rather than competition. For example, success in a cardiac arrest simulation might be measured by specific criteria such as maintaining the correct rate and depth of chest compressions and ensuring learners meet predefined standards.

5. **Student-Oriented Instruction**

    At its core, ADDIE is designed to prioritize the learner. Objectives are articulated in terms of what the learner can do, and instruction is framed around student activities rather than instructor performance. This aligns with adult learning principles, recognizing that learners actively participate in their education. For example, a scenario might include interactive decision-making elements where learners choose how to manage a deteriorating patient, promoting engagement and autonomy.

6. **Shared Goals and Transparency**

    ADDIE promotes clear communication of instructional goals to both the learner and the instructor. This ensures that all participants understand the objectives and when those objectives have been achieved. In healthcare simulation, this might involve providing learners with a checklist of expected competencies and using post-simulation debriefing to confirm whether those competencies were demonstrated. Transparency fosters accountability and helps learners track their progress.

7. **Accountability for System Design**

    A critical principle of ADDIE is recognizing that if learners fail to meet objectives, the fault may lie with the instructional system rather than the student. This concept underscores the iterative nature of the ADDIE model: the system must be re-evaluated and adjusted until it effectively meets learner needs. For example, suppose learners consistently struggle with a scenario. In that case, facilitators might revisit the Design phase to ensure the objectives are clear or modify the Development phase to include more realistic cues.

The Impact of Key Concepts

These guiding principles make ADDIE a robust and reliable framework for instructional design. By ensuring instruction is relevant, targeted, and measurable, ADDIE helps create educational experiences that are effective and empowering for learners. In healthcare simulation, where the stakes are high, and the skills learned directly impact patient outcomes, these principles provide the structure needed to deliver meaningful and transformative training.

Adhering to these concepts, the ADDIE model ensures learners acquire the knowledge, skills, and attitudes they need to excel in their roles. Through its commitment to learner-centered design, transparency, and accountability, ADDIE continues to shape the future of education and training in healthcare and beyond.

Why ADDIE Works in Healthcare Simulation

Healthcare simulation is a unique educational modality, blending the art of teaching with healthcare science. The ADDIE model's systematic approach makes it particularly well-suited to this field for several reasons:

- **Ensuring a Learner-Centered Approach**
  At its core, ADDIE emphasizes understanding and addressing learners' needs. In healthcare simulation, this means designing relevant, challenging scenarios that align with the learners' level of expertise. For example, a simulation for novice nursing students might focus on basic skills, while one for experienced clinicians might address advanced decision-making in complex cases (Rosen et al., 2008).

- **Aligning Simulation Objectives with Clinical Goals**
  Effective healthcare simulations are grounded in real-world clinical objectives. The ADDIE model ensures that these objectives are clearly defined during the Analysis phase and carried through each subsequent phase. This alignment enhances the relevance and impact of the simulation, ensuring that learners can transfer their skills to actual clinical practice (Fanning & Gaba, 2007).

For instance, a simulation to reduce hospital-acquired infections might focus on proper hand hygiene, sterile techniques, and teamwork during procedures. The training becomes practical and meaningful by aligning the simulation objectives with this broader clinical goal.

- **Fostering Continuous Improvement**
  The iterative nature of ADDIE allows for ongoing refinement. By incorporating evaluation feedback, instructional designers can enhance the simulation's effectiveness over time. This is particularly valuable in healthcare, where standards and practices continually evolve (Jeffries, 2012).

- **Promoting Interprofessional Collaboration**
  Healthcare simulation often involves diverse teams, including physicians, nurses, and allied health professionals. The ADDIE model's structured approach facilitates collaboration among these stakeholders, ensuring that the simulation meets the needs of all participants (Zigmont et al., 2011).

Conclusion

The ADDIE model is more than just a framework; it is a powerful tool for creating meaningful and impactful educational experiences. Educators and instructional designers can fully harness its potential by understanding its origins, core elements, and unique advantages in healthcare simulation. In the upcoming chapters, we will examine each phase of ADDIE, and you will acquire the knowledge and tools necessary to design, develop, and deliver simulations that truly make a difference.

Key Takeaways

1. The ADDIE model provides a structured and systematic approach to instructional design, making it adaptable and effective across various fields, including healthcare simulation.

2. Each phase—Analyze, Design, Develop, Implement, and Evaluate—plays a critical role in ensuring the success of educational initiatives.
3. ADDIE highlights a learner-centered approach in healthcare simulation, aligning objectives with clinical goals and promoting interprofessional collaboration.
4. The model's iterative nature allows for continuous improvement, ensuring that simulations remain relevant and impactful in the ever-evolving healthcare landscape.
5. By understanding and applying ADDIE, educators can design simulations that teach technical skills and promote teamwork, communication, and critical thinking.

Reflection

As we reflect on the ADDIE model, it becomes clear why it has endured as a cornerstone of instructional design. Its adaptability and focus on systematic planning make it an ideal framework for creating impactful educational experiences in healthcare. The Analyze phase ensures that the foundation is strong, the Design and Develop phases bring creativity and precision, and the Implement and Evaluate phases close the loop by ensuring effectiveness and fostering improvement.

For educators and designers in healthcare simulation, ADDIE is more than a process; it is a mindset. By embracing its principles, we can create simulations that not only prepare learners for the complexities of clinical practice but also inspire confidence and competence. As you move forward, consider how the principles of ADDIE can inform your own work, turning challenges into opportunities for growth and excellence.

References

Allen, W. C. (2006). Overview and evolution of the ADDIE training system. Advances in Developing Human Resources, 8(4), 430-441.

Allen, W. C. (2006). Overview and evolution of the ADDIE training system. Advances in Developing Human Resources, 8(4), 430–441. https://doi.org/10.1177/1523422306292942

Bloom, B. S. (1956). Taxonomy of educational objectives: The classification of educational goals. Longman.

Branch, R. M. (2009). Instructional design: The ADDIE approach. Springer Science & Business Media.

Dick, W., Carey, L., & Carey, J. O. (2005). The systematic design of instruction (6th ed.). Pearson.

Fanning, R. M., & Gaba, D. M. (2007). The role of debriefing in simulation-based learning. Simulation in Healthcare, 2(2), 115-125.

Gagné, R. M., Wager, W. W., Golas, K. C., & Keller, J. M. (2005). Principles of instructional design (5th ed.). Wadsworth/Thomson Learning.

Hodell, C. (2016). ISD: From the ground up: A concise introduction to instructional design (4th ed.). American Society for Training and Development.

Jeffries, P. R. (2012). Simulation in nursing education: From conceptualization to evaluation. National League for Nursing.

Kirkpatrick, D. L., & Kirkpatrick, J. D. (2006). Evaluating training programs: The four levels. Berrett-Koehler Publishers.

Morrison, G. R., Ross, S. M., Kalman, H. K., & Kemp, J. E. (2013). Designing effective instruction (7th ed.). Wiley.

Reigeluth, C. M. (1999). Instructional-design theories and models: A new paradigm of instructional theory (Vol. 2). Routledge.

Reiser, R. A., & Dempsey, J. V. (2017). Trends and issues in instructional design and technology (4th ed.). Pearson.

Rosen, M. A., Salas, E., Silvestri, S., Wu, T. S., & Lazzara, E. H. (2008). Promoting teamwork: An event-based approach to simulation-based teamwork training for emergency medicine residents. Academic Emergency Medicine, 15(11), 1190-1198.

Zigmont, J. J., Kappus, L. J., & Sudikoff, S. N. (2011). The 3D model of debriefing: Defusing, discovering, and deepening. Seminars in Perinatology, 35(2), 52-58.

"Anyone who stops learning is old, whether at twenty or eighty. Anyone who keeps learning stays young."
— Henry Ford

Chapter 2
Analyze Phase in Healthcare Simulation

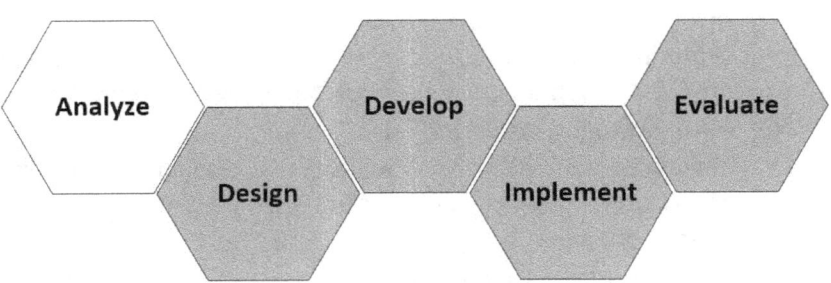

Introduction to the Analyze Phase

The Analyze phase is the foundation of the ADDIE model, serving as the cornerstone upon which all other phases are built. In healthcare simulation, this phase is particularly critical. It involves identifying training needs, defining the learner population, and setting clear, measurable goals and objectives. By carefully analyzing these elements, educators and instructional designers ensure that simulations address real-world challenges and meet the specific needs of learners.

Healthcare environments are complex and ever evolving, making it essential to pinpoint gaps in clinical knowledge, skills, and performance. The Analyze phase ensures that the simulations designed are relevant, effective, and capable of fostering meaningful learning experiences. This chapter explores the essential steps of the Analyze phase, providing practical strategies and examples to guide your efforts.

Identifying Training Needs

Assessing Gaps in Clinical Skills and Knowledge

The first step in the Analyze phase is assessing clinical skills and knowledge gaps. This process involves identifying where learners lack proficiency or confidence and pinpointing systemic issues that affect patient care.

Methods for Identifying Training Needs:

- **Observation:**
  Shadowing healthcare professionals in clinical settings can reveal gaps in practice or workflow inefficiencies.
- **Interviews and Focus Groups:**
  Engaging with learners, supervisors, and other stakeholders provides insights into perceived challenges and unmet needs.
- **Performance Data Analysis:**
  Reviewing metrics such as medical errors, patient outcomes, or procedural success rates can help identify areas for improvement.
- **Competency Assessments:**
  Administering tests or simulations to evaluate learners' skills and knowledge provides objective data on performance gaps.

For example, a hospital might notice a high incidence of medication errors in their ICU. A deeper analysis could reveal that these errors stem from poor communication during handoffs. Identifying this need allows the organization to design a simulation that improves communication protocols.

Aligning Needs with Organizational Goals

While identifying individual learner needs is critical, aligning training efforts with broader organizational goals is equally important.

Healthcare organizations often have strategic objectives, such as reducing hospital-acquired infections or improving patient satisfaction scores. Simulations should support these goals, ensuring that training efforts have a tangible impact on organizational performance.

Defining Learners

Understanding Audience Demographics

Defining the learner population is a vital aspect of the Analyze phase. Healthcare simulation often involves diverse audiences, ranging from medical students and nurses to seasoned clinicians and administrative staff. Understanding your learners' demographics, professional roles, and experience levels helps tailor simulations to their specific needs.

Key Factors to Consider:

1. **Professional Backgrounds:** What clinical roles do learners occupy? For example, a simulation designed for nurses will differ from one aimed at physicians.
2. **Experience Levels:** Are learners novices, intermediates, or experts in their field?
3. **Cultural and Linguistic Considerations:** Ensure simulations are inclusive and address the diverse backgrounds of participants.

Learning Preferences and Styles

People learn in different ways, and understanding your audience's learning preferences can enhance the effectiveness of your simulations. Some learners prefer hands-on, experiential learning, while others thrive on structured, theoretical approaches. Gathering insights into learning preferences through surveys or discussions helps shape the simulation design.

Example: A group of paramedics participating in a trauma simulation might benefit from a highly interactive, scenario-based approach. In contrast, administrative staff undergoing a simulation on patient communication might require a more discussion-focused format.

Setting Goals and Objectives

<u>Establishing Clear and Measurable Outcomes</u>

Setting goals and objectives is the final and most crucial step of the analysis phase. Goals provide the overarching purpose of the simulation, while objectives break this purpose down into specific, measurable outcomes. Well-defined objectives ensure that simulations remain focused and effective, offering a clear benchmark for success.

SMART Objectives:

1. **Specific:** Clearly state what learners will achieve.
2. **Measurable:** Include criteria for evaluating success.
3. **Achievable:** Ensure objectives are realistic given the resources and constraints.
4. **Relevant:** Align objectives with learner needs and organizational goals.
5. **Time-Bound:** Specify a timeframe for achieving the objectives.

Example of a Simulation Objective: "By the end of the simulation, learners will demonstrate the ability to perform adult CPR according to current guidelines with 90% accuracy."

<u>Terminal and Enabling Objectives</u>

In the ADDIE model, **terminal** and **enabling objectives** are crucial in defining the scope and structure of learning experiences. Together, they create a roadmap for instructional design, ensuring that learners progress from foundational knowledge and skills to achieving overarching educational goals.

What Are Terminal and Enabling Objectives?

Terminal Objectives
Terminal objectives are high-level goals that define what learners should be able to accomplish by the end of a training or instructional

program. They broadly describe the desired performance outcomes and align with the overall purpose of the simulation or curriculum. These objectives are typically tied to key competencies or standards, such as those established by the Accreditation Council for Graduate Medical Education (ACGME) or the American Association of Colleges of Nursing (AACN) Essentials (Jeffries, 2012).

Enabling Objectives
Enabling objectives are the smaller, more specific steps learners must master to achieve the terminal objective. They break down complex skills or knowledge into manageable components, providing a structured pathway for learning. These objectives often focus on foundational tasks or prerequisite knowledge that builds toward the terminal objective (Gagné et al., 2005).

How They Work Together
The relationship between terminal and enabling objectives can be visualized as a hierarchy:
Terminal Objective: The ultimate goal learners are working toward.
Enabling Objectives: The incremental steps that support the achievement of the terminal objective.

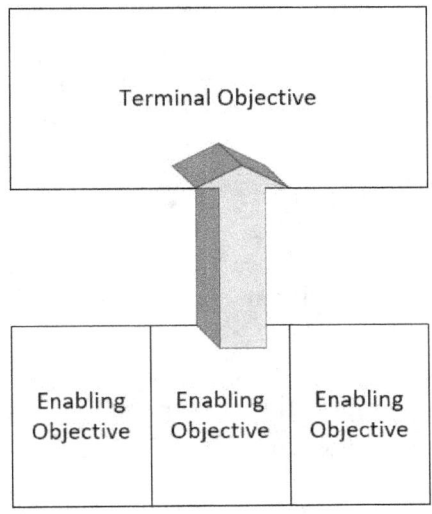

This structure ensures logical progression, enabling learners to systematically develop the necessary skills and knowledge.

Examples of Terminal and Enabling Objectives

Example 1: Communication in Healthcare Teams

Terminal Objective:
Demonstrate effective team communication during a high-pressure clinical scenario, using closed-loop communication and clear role delegation.
(Aligned with ACGME competency: Interpersonal and Communication Skills)

Enabling Objectives:
- Identify barriers to effective team communication in healthcare settings.
- Practice closed-loop communication techniques in low-stress simulations.
- Use SBAR (Situation, Background, Assessment, Recommendation) to convey critical information during patient handoffs.

Example 2: Managing a Cardiac Arrest

Terminal Objective:
Perform as the team leader in a simulated cardiac arrest, adhering to Advanced Cardiac Life Support (ACLS) guidelines to ensure optimal patient care outcomes.
(Aligned with LCME standard: Patient Care)

Enabling Objectives:
- Recognize signs of cardiac arrest and initiate the ACLS algorithm within 30 seconds.
- Direct team members to perform chest compressions, ventilation, and defibrillation appropriately.
- Interpret electrocardiogram (ECG) findings to guide treatment decisions.

Example 3: Medication Safety

Terminal Objective:
Safely administer medications during a simulated patient care scenario, following the "five rights" of medication administration. *(Aligned with AACN Essential: Patient-Centered Care)*

Enabling Objectives:
- Verify patient identity and match it to the prescribed medication order.
- Calculate correct medication dosages based on patient weight and clinical guidelines.
- Identify and address potential contraindications before administering medications.

Benefits of Using Terminal and Enabling Objectives
- **Clarity and Focus**
  Terminal objectives provide learners with a clear understanding of what they are expected to achieve by the end of the program, while enabling objectives help them focus on mastering the necessary skills and knowledge incrementally.

- **Alignment with Standards**
  By linking objectives to professional standards and competencies (e.g., ACGME milestones, AACN Essentials), educators ensure that training aligns with industry expectations and enhances real-world readiness.

- **Enhanced Assessment**
  Terminal objectives support summative evaluation, measuring whether learners have achieved the program's goals. Enabling objectives facilitate formative assessments, providing opportunities for feedback and improvement during the learning process (Gagné et al., 2005).

Terminal and enabling objectives are foundational elements of the ADDIE model, ensuring that instructional design is structured, purposeful, and aligned with desired outcomes. By breaking down complex goals into achievable steps, they enable learners to build competence progressively and achieve success in healthcare simulation and beyond.

The ABCD Method of Writing Objectives

Audience — Who is the intended audience?

Behavior — Using an action verb, identify what the audience will be doing

Condition — What situation or environment will the audience perform the behavior?

Degree of Mastery (aka Standard) — How will you measure success?

Clear and measurable objectives are the foundation of effective learning experiences. The **ABCD method** offers a simple and structured way to craft objectives that ensure both clarity and focus.

Each component in the ABCD framework addresses a key aspect of what learners are expected to achieve.

A - Audience
The first step is identifying **who** the objective is targeting. This is the learner or participant. Being specific about the audience allows you to focus on their unique needs, ensuring the objective is tailored appropriately. For example, "The student will..." or "The participant will..."

B - Behavior
The behavior defines **what** the learner will do. It should be an observable and measurable action, often described using action verbs like "identify," "describe," "demonstrate," or "analyze." This ensures there is no ambiguity in what the learner is expected to accomplish. For example, "The student will identify the key components of a simulation scenario."

C - Condition
The condition specifies the **circumstances** under which the behavior will occur. This might include the tools, resources, or environment provided to the learner. For instance, "Using a simulated patient scenario," or "Given access to a data set..." Adding conditions gives the objective context, making it more realistic and achievable.

D - Degree
The degree outlines the **criteria for success** or the expected level of performance. This could involve accuracy, speed, or completeness. For example, "with 90% accuracy" or "within 10 minutes." Including a degree makes the objective measurable, allowing educators to assess whether the learner has achieved the desired outcome.

Putting It All Together

Here's an example of the ABCD method in action:

Audience: The nursing student
Behavior: Will demonstrate proper handwashing techniques

Condition: Using a simulated hospital sink and soap
Degree: Following all five steps of hand hygiene according to WHO guidelines

Objective: *The nursing student will demonstrate proper handwashing techniques using a simulated hospital sink and soap, following all five steps of hand hygiene according to WHO guidelines.*

The ABCD method ensures that objectives are specific, measurable, and relevant, making them a cornerstone of effective instructional design. Educators and trainers can align their goals with desired outcomes by applying this framework, ultimately enhancing the learning experience.

The objectives could be written and look like CABD instead.

Here's an example of the CABD method in action:

Condition: Using a simulated hospital sink and soap
Audience: The nursing student
Behavior: Will demonstrate proper handwashing techniques
Degree: Following all five steps of hand hygiene according to WHO guidelines

Objective: *Using a simulated hospital sink and soap, the nursing student will demonstrate proper handwashing techniques by following all five steps of hand hygiene according to WHO guidelines.*

Linking Objectives to Outcomes

The power of well-crafted objectives in healthcare simulation cannot be overstated. Objectives serve as the simulation's guiding stars, ensuring every activity, scenario, and debrief aligns to improve patient care. They transform abstract intentions into tangible, actionable targets that guide educators and facilitators and set clear learner expectations.

Linking Objectives to Outcomes

Objectives must be meticulously linked to desired outcomes to create purposeful and strategic simulations. Consider a simulation designed to enhance teamwork within surgical teams. Without clear objectives, the simulation might meander, haphazardly addressing issues. However, when objectives are explicitly tied to outcomes—such as improving communication under stress, enhancing role clarity during emergencies, and fostering effective decision-making—the simulation becomes targeted and impactful.

For example, an objective to "demonstrate closed-loop communication during high-pressure scenarios" directly ties to the outcome of reducing communication errors. Learners participating in such a simulation experience a clear connection between their performance and the real-world challenges they will face. During the debriefing, facilitators can explicitly link observed behaviors to the stated objectives, helping participants internalize lessons and apply them in their practice. This alignment not only improves the quality of the simulation but also maximizes its impact on patient care outcomes.

Linking Objectives to Competencies and Standards
In healthcare, competencies and professional standards provide a foundation for designing simulations that reflect industry expectations. By aligning objectives with recognized frameworks such as the Accreditation Council for Graduate Medical Education (ACGME) competencies, the Commission on Collegiate Nursing Education (CCNE) standards, the American Association of Colleges of Nursing (AACN) Essentials, or the Liaison Committee on Medical Education (LCME) standards, simulations can ensure relevance, rigor, and alignment with professional benchmarks.

For instance, if the ACGME competency in "Interpersonal and Communication Skills" is targeted, simulation objectives might include:
- "Demonstrate effective handoff communication using SBAR (Situation, Background, Assessment, Recommendation)."
- "Engage in collaborative decision-making with a multidisciplinary team."

Similarly, a simulation designed for nursing students might link to the CCNE standard emphasizing "Patient-Centered Care," with objectives such as:

- "Develop a care plan based on patient preferences and evidence-based practices."
- "Apply culturally competent communication techniques during patient interactions."

Learners meet simulation-specific goals and progress toward broader professional standards by connecting objectives to such competencies. This alignment ensures that simulations prepare learners for isolated tasks and holistic, competency-based excellence in their fields.

Limiting Objectives in Simulation

When designing simulations, particularly in healthcare or other high-stakes industries, it can be tempting to cram as many objectives as possible into a single scenario. After all, the more objectives covered, the more "efficient" the simulation might seem. However, overloading a simulation with too many goals can dilute its effectiveness, overwhelm participants, and make assessment challenging. Limiting the number of objectives is a strategic approach that enhances both learning outcomes and the overall simulation experience.

Enhancing Focus and Clarity

One of the primary benefits of narrowing the number of objectives is the focus it provides to both facilitators and participants. A simulation with a manageable number of objectives allows participants to dedicate their mental resources to mastering specific skills or concepts without feeling overburdened. For example, in a healthcare simulation, concentrating on two or three key learning points—such as effective communication during a crisis and adherence to protocol—ensures participants can thoroughly practice and reflect on these critical areas.

On the facilitator's side, a reduced set of objectives streamlines the design, execution, and debriefing processes. With fewer goals to track, instructors can focus on observing participants' performance and providing targeted feedback that aligns with the primary learning outcomes.

Supporting Cognitive Load Theory

Research in cognitive psychology, particularly Cognitive Load Theory, underscores the importance of managing the mental demands placed on learners (Sweller, 1988). Overloading participants with multiple objectives can exceed their cognitive capacity, especially when navigating a high-fidelity simulation's complexities. This often leads to superficial engagement with the objectives and a failure to retain key lessons. Limiting the scope of the simulation objectives ensures participants can effectively process, retain, and apply the knowledge or skills being targeted.

Improving Measurability and Assessment

Simulations are often used as assessment tools, whether for evaluating clinical competencies, decision-making, or teamwork. However, assessing participant performance becomes increasingly challenging when there are too many objectives. A limited set of clearly defined objectives allows facilitators to focus their assessments on specific behaviors or outcomes. For instance, if the objective is to practice effective team communication, facilitators can observe and evaluate specific interactions, such as closed-loop communication or clear delegation of tasks, rather than trying to track multiple unrelated behaviors simultaneously.

Facilitating Debriefing

Debriefing is arguably the most critical component of any simulation, allowing participants to reflect on their actions and internalize lessons learned. The debriefing process becomes more structured and meaningful when simulations include manageable objectives. Facilitators can guide discussions around the key objectives, ensuring participants leave with a clear understanding of what they did well and where they need improvement. In contrast, simulations with excessive objectives often result in fragmented debriefing sessions, where important lessons are overlooked or not given adequate attention.

Encouraging Iterative Learning

Finally, by limiting the number of objectives, simulations can be designed as part of a broader curriculum that allows for iterative learning. Participants can engage in multiple scenarios, each with a specific focus, progressively building on their skills. For example, one simulation might focus on mastering technical procedures, while a subsequent scenario emphasizes leadership under pressure. This incremental approach promotes deeper learning and helps participants develop a more comprehensive skill set.

In summary, limiting the number of objectives in a simulation maximizes its educational impact by enhancing focus, supporting cognitive load management, improving assessment, facilitating effective debriefing, and encouraging iterative learning. By resisting the urge to cover "everything" in a single simulation, facilitators can create targeted, meaningful experiences that lead to lasting behavioral and cognitive change.

Its Ok for Simulations Not to Meet All the Objectives

A common misconception in simulation-based learning is that every objective must be fully met during the scenario. While achieving objectives in real-time is ideal, it's important to recognize that learning doesn't end when the scenario does. The true power of simulation lies in its ability to foster reflective discussion during the debriefing process. When learners do not meet all the objectives in the scenario, facilitators can guide them toward understanding the intent of those objectives during the debrief, turning missed opportunities into valuable teaching moments.

Debriefing Bridges the Gap

Debriefing is the cornerstone of simulation-based education, allowing learners to process their performance, discuss their actions, and connect their experiences to the intended objectives. If participants struggle with a particular objective—such as managing effective communication under pressure or performing a psychomotor skill like chest compressions at the correct rate—the debrief becomes an opportunity to explore what happened, why it happened, and how it can be improved.

Through this reflective process, learners often achieve the intent of the objective by identifying their gaps and articulating how they might address those gaps in future scenarios or real-life situations. For instance, if a learner struggles to properly execute a procedural skill during a simulation, discussing the key steps, common errors, and troubleshooting strategies in the debrief can provide the clarity needed for mastery. In this way, the debrief serves as an extension of the learning process, reinforcing the objectives and ensuring that the learners still meet the educational goals.

Psychomotor Objectives and Iterative Learning

Psychomotor objectives, such as performing a clinical skill or utilizing equipment correctly, are particularly well-suited to this approach. These objectives often require repetitive practice and feedback to achieve proficiency, and it's unrealistic to expect mastery in a single attempt. Suppose learners do not fully meet a psychomotor objective during a scenario. In that case, facilitators can use the debrief to review the correct technique, discuss areas for improvement, and encourage participants to try again.

Re-running the scenario or incorporating the same objective into a future simulation provides learners with another opportunity to practice and solidify their skills. For example, suppose a learner fails to establish IV access during a scenario. In that case, the facilitator can provide immediate feedback during the debrief and either allow the learner to retry the skill in a subsequent run of the same scenario or embed the skill into a different scenario. This iterative process builds confidence, muscle memory, and competence over time.

Building Resilience and Adaptive Thinking

Allowing learners to struggle with objectives during a scenario also has the added benefit of teaching resilience and adaptive thinking. In real-life situations, not everything goes as planned. Simulations that present challenges or highlight areas for improvement prepare learners to adapt to unforeseen circumstances. When objectives are not met in the scenario but are thoroughly discussed and understood during the debrief, learners are better equipped to handle similar challenges in the future.

Aligning with Educational Goals

Ultimately, the goal of simulation is not perfection but progression. By emphasizing the learning process rather than the outcome of a single scenario, facilitators create an environment where mistakes are viewed as opportunities for growth. This approach helps learners feel less intimidated by their errors and more willing to engage in meaningful discussions about how to improve.

It's perfectly okay—and often beneficial—for simulations not to meet all objectives during the scenario. The debrief provides an invaluable platform for achieving the intent of those objectives through discussion, reflection, and feedback. Repeated practice across scenarios helps learners build proficiency and confidence for psychomotor objectives. This flexible approach ensures that learners grasp the material and develop the resilience and adaptability they need for real-world success.

Maximizing Evaluation and Improvement

When objectives are linked to outcomes and competencies, they enhance evaluation efforts by providing a clear framework for assessing simulation effectiveness. Objectives that are SMART (Specific, Measurable, Achievable, Relevant, and Time-bound) enable educators to evaluate performance with precision:

- Did participants demonstrate the desired behaviors?
- Were clinical competencies appropriately applied?
- Did the simulation address relevant standards, such as those outlined by the AACN Essentials or ACGME milestones?

For example, a simulation aligned with the LCME standard on "Medical Knowledge" might include an objective to "apply evidence-based diagnostic criteria to recognize early signs of sepsis." Evaluation tools like checklists and rubrics can then assess whether learners met this objective, offering actionable insights for refining future simulations.

Creating Transformative Simulations
By linking objectives to outcomes, competencies, and standards, healthcare simulations become more than training exercises—they evolve into transformative experiences. Learners see the direct relevance of their actions, not only to immediate tasks but also to the broader demands of their professional roles. This alignment prepares them to navigate the complexities of real-world patient care with confidence, competence, and a commitment to continuous improvement.

What To Do If There Isn't Time for an In-Depth Analysis

While the Analysis phase is essential for designing effective healthcare simulations, there are situations where time constraints or urgent needs make a comprehensive analysis challenging. Healthcare settings often demand rapid responses to emerging training needs, such as addressing new protocols, technologies, or critical incidents. In these cases, a streamlined approach to analysis can still ensure the simulation meets its objectives without compromising quality.

1. **Conduct a Rapid Needs Assessment**
   When time is limited, prioritize a focused and concise assessment of training needs.

   <u>Gather Input Quickly:</u>

Use brief surveys, interviews, or focus groups with key stakeholders (e.g., managers, clinicians, or educators) to identify the most pressing performance gaps.

Leverage Existing Data:
Use available information, such as patient safety reports, clinical error trends, or learner feedback, to pinpoint areas needing improvement.

Prioritize Key Goals:
Instead of a comprehensive list of all potential objectives, focus on the "must-have" outcomes.

Example: Instead of analyzing every aspect of a surgical team's performance, focus on immediate issues like communication breakdowns in high-stakes procedures.

2. **Use Pre-Existing Resources**
   In time-sensitive situations, don't reinvent the wheel.

   Adapt Existing Simulations:
   Modify previously developed scenarios to suit the current need. For instance, a simulation designed for cardiac arrest can be tailored to focus on specific areas like medication administration or teamwork.

   Utilize Established Frameworks:
   Employ standardized protocols, such as Advanced Cardiac Life Support (ACLS) guidelines, as a foundation for your simulation objectives.

   Example: If the goal is to address ventilator management for COVID-19 patients, adapt an existing respiratory care simulation by emphasizing new protocols or challenges unique to the pandemic.

3. **Engage Subject Matter Experts (SMEs)**
   SMEs can provide critical insights to fast-track the analysis process.

Collaborate with Clinicians:
Nurses, physicians, and other healthcare professionals with hands-on experience can quickly identify training gaps and priorities.

Ask Targeted Questions:
Concentrate on the areas where learners face the most difficulty, identify common errors, and determine what new practices should be adopted.

Example: A brief conversation with an ICU nurse manager might reveal that staff need immediate training on operating new infusion pumps, allowing you to focus the simulation on this critical skill.

4. **Start Small and Iterate**
When time is limited, create a minimally viable simulation and improve it gradually.

Focus on Core Objectives:
Select one or two essential skills or behaviors to emphasize in the simulation.

Plan for Feedback and Iteration:
The first implementation should serve as training and a way to gather data for further refinement.

Example: Launch a basic scenario on emergency intubation techniques and enhance it later with more complex variables, such as difficult airway management.

5. **Use Simulated or Mock Data**
Use simulated data or assumptions based on typical performance gaps if direct learner data is unavailable.

Estimate Learner Needs:
Use general industry trends or previous experience to hypothesize areas of focus.

Validate Assumptions Quickly:
Before full deployment, run the scenario with a small group to confirm the relevance of the objectives.

Example: If no specific learner data is available, assume that junior nurses might need refresher training on medication administration safety based on broader industry findings.

6. **Align With Broader Organizational Goals**
When time prevents detailed learner analysis, align the simulation's objectives with overarching organizational goals.

Focus on Key Metrics:
Target areas tied to patient safety, compliance, or accreditation requirements.

Engage Leadership:
Consult organizational leaders to ensure the simulation supports high-priority initiatives.

Example: If reducing central line infections is a hospital priority, create a simulation focusing on sterile techniques and team communication during central line insertions.

7. **Document What You Can**
Even in a time crunch, document the rationale behind your decisions.

Create a Brief Analysis Summary:
Record the key issues, objectives, and resources identified.

Use This as a Baseline:
This documentation can guide post-simulation evaluations and help refine future iterations.

Example: A quick note stating, "Simulation addresses increased medication errors identified in recent incident reports," provides clarity and direction for future efforts.

Balancing Speed and Quality

While a comprehensive analysis is ideal, these strategies allow for effective, targeted simulations even when time is limited. Focusing on immediate needs, leveraging existing resources, and involving SMEs, educators, and instructional designers can ensure the simulation remains impactful and relevant. The key is to remain flexible, prioritize critical outcomes, and view the initial effort as part of an iterative process that can be refined over time.

Case Study: Analyzing Needs for a Simulation on Sepsis Management

Scenario: A regional hospital identifies sepsis management as a critical area for improvement. Data reveals that delayed recognition and treatment of sepsis have led to increased mortality rates.

Analyze Phase Steps:

1. **Identify Training Needs:**
   - Observations reveal that staff often fail to recognize early signs of sepsis.
   - Interviews with clinicians highlight confusion around sepsis protocols.
2. **Define Learners:**
   - The primary audience includes nurses and junior physicians.
   - A secondary audience involves administrative staff responsible for triaging patients.
3. **Set Goals and Objectives:**
   - **Goal:** Improve the early identification and treatment of sepsis.
   - **Objectives:**
     - Learners will correctly identify the early signs of sepsis in 90% of cases.

- Learners will demonstrate adherence to the hospital's sepsis treatment protocol during simulations.

This structured approach ensures that the subsequent simulation effectively addresses the identified gaps and supports the hospital's goal of reducing sepsis-related mortality.

Detailed Role of Stakeholders in the Analysis Phase

The Analysis phase is foundational in the ADDIE model, setting the stage for designing and delivering impactful healthcare simulation programs. During this phase, the involvement of key stakeholders ensures that the training program aligns with organizational goals, addresses learner needs, and utilizes available resources effectively. Each stakeholder plays a distinct role in contributing expertise, insights, and support, making their participation essential for a comprehensive analysis.

Key Stakeholders and Their Roles

Stakeholder	Role in Analysis Phase	Contributions
Educators	Provide insights into learner performance and identify gaps in knowledge, skills, and attitudes.	- Identify areas where learners struggle. - Highlight priorities for simulation scenarios. - Propose focus areas for learning objectives.
Facilitators	Bridge theory and practice by highlighting logistical needs and learner challenges.	- Share common learner behaviors. - Identify logistical needs such as equipment and time requirements. - Provide input on feasibility of identified needs.

Administrators	Ensure alignment of analysis with organizational goals, budget, and resource constraints.	- Define organizational priorities for training. - Facilitate collaboration between departments. - Approve funding for analysis-related activities.
Subject Matter Experts (SMEs)	Contribute clinical expertise to define critical knowledge and validate identified gaps.	- Validate clinical relevance of gaps. - Provide data on best practices and standards. - Confirm accuracy of proposed learning focus areas.
Learners	Share firsthand challenges and preferences, helping to pinpoint areas requiring improvement.	- Participate in focus groups or surveys. - Highlight skills or tasks they feel underprepared for. - Share preferred learning styles.

Collaborative Effort for Comprehensive Analysis

Effective analysis relies on collaboration among these stakeholders to create a well-rounded understanding of the training needs. By combining the perspectives of educators, facilitators, administrators, SMEs, and learners, the Analysis phase ensures that the simulation program:

- Addresses real-world clinical challenges.
- Aligns with organizational priorities and professional standards.
- Provides meaningful, engaging, and practical learning experiences.

Defining the roles of stakeholders during the Analysis phase ensures a robust foundation for healthcare simulation programs. Each stakeholder brings unique insights that contribute to a comprehensive understanding of training needs, ensuring the program is relevant, effective, and aligned with broader organizational goals. This collaborative approach sets the stage for successfully implementing the ADDIE model in healthcare education.

Analysis Phase: Inputs and Outputs

The Analysis phase is the foundation of the ADDIE model. In this phase, the instructional designer identifies the problem, defines the goals, and determines the needs of the learners and the organization. This phase is critical because it sets the direction for the subsequent phases, ensuring that the training program aligns with specific objectives and addresses real gaps in knowledge, skills, or behaviors.

Inputs to the Analysis Phase

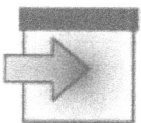

Inputs are the information, resources, and tools needed to conduct a thorough analysis. These inputs provide the data and insights required to define the scope and purpose of the instructional intervention.

Organizational Needs
- Strategic goals, priorities, and challenges that the training program must address.

    Example: A hospital aiming to reduce medication errors by 20% within a year.

Stakeholder Input
- Perspectives from administrators, educators, clinicians, and learners to identify training priorities.

    Example: Nursing staff reporting frequent challenges with IV medication administration.

Job and Task Analysis
- A breakdown of tasks, responsibilities, and competencies required for a specific role.

Example: Identifying key steps in managing a sepsis patient, such as early recognition and intervention.

Learner Demographics and Characteristics
- Information about the target audience, including:
    - Job roles and levels of experience.
    - Learning preferences and prior knowledge.

Example: A team of novice nurses needing foundational training in emergency response.

Data Collection Methods
- Tools and strategies to gather insights, such as:
    - Surveys and questionnaires.
    - Focus groups or interviews.
    - Performance reports or incident reviews.

Example: Reviewing error logs to identify patterns in medication administration mistakes.

Constraints and Resources
- Limitations and assets, such as:
    - Budget, time, and personnel.
    - Available equipment, technology, and training space.

Example: Limited access to high-fidelity mannequins for simulations.

Outputs of the Analysis Phase

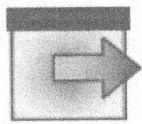

Outputs are the results or deliverables that emerge from the analysis phase. These outputs provide a clear roadmap for the Design phase, ensuring that the training program is aligned with learner and organizational needs.

Defined Learning Needs

- A summary of the gaps in knowledge, skills, or attitudes that the training must address.

    Example: Nurses need to improve their ability to perform accurate medication dosage calculations under stress.

Target Audience Profile
- A detailed description of the learners, including their roles, experience levels, and learning preferences.

    Example: A group of 20 ICU nurses with 1–3 years of experience requiring simulation-based training on crisis management.

Learning Objectives
- High-level objectives that specify what learners should know or be able to do after the training.

    Example: "Demonstrate closed-loop communication during a cardiac arrest scenario."

Scope of Training
- A clear definition of what the training will and will not cover.

    Example: The program will focus on team communication and technical skills for managing sepsis, excluding unrelated procedures like wound care.

Data-Driven Insights
- Key findings from surveys, focus groups, and performance reports.

    Example: Incident reports show that 75% of medication errors occurred during shift changes.

Constraints and Assumptions
- Identification of limitations and initial strategies to address them.

Example: A limited budget may require low-fidelity simulations instead of advanced VR technology.

Analysis Report
- A formal document summarizing findings, goals, and recommendations.

Example: A report outlining the need for interdisciplinary team training in emergency room triage procedures.

Analysis Phase	
Inputs	**Outputs (Deliverables)**
☐ Organizational Need ☐ Stakeholder Input ☐ Job & Task Analysis ☐ Learner Demographics & Characteristics ☐ Data Collection Methods ☐ Constraints & Resources	☐ Defined Learning Needs ☐ Target Audience Profile ☐ Learning Objectives ☐ Scope of Training ☐ Data-driven Insights ☐ Constraints & Assumptions ☐ Analysis Report

<u>How Inputs Lead to Outputs</u>

The success of the Analysis phase relies on effectively transforming inputs into actionable outputs. For instance:

Input: Surveys reveal that learners struggle with prioritizing tasks during emergencies.

Output: A learning objective is created: "Prioritize life-saving interventions based on patient condition during a trauma scenario."

The analysis phase systematically processes inputs, ensuring the training program is relevant, targeted, and aligned with measurable goals.

The Analysis phase serves as the blueprint for the entire ADDIE process. By identifying the instructional needs through robust inputs and translating them into actionable outputs, this phase ensures that the training program is effective and aligned with organizational and learner priorities. This clarity is essential for creating simulations that are not only educational but also transformative in improving real-world outcomes.

Analysis Phase:
Questions to Ask
1. What performance gaps or issues are we trying to address?
2. What specific skills, knowledge, or behaviors are learners lacking?
3. What evidence supports the need for this training (e.g., incident reports, performance reviews, patient safety data)?
4. Are external factors driving this simulation's need (e.g., regulatory changes, new technologies, or protocols)?
5. Who are the target learners, and what are their roles in the organization?
6. What are the learners' current level of knowledge, skills, and experience?
7. Are there varying levels of expertise within the learner group that must be addressed?
8. What learning preferences or styles do these learners typically exhibit?
9. Are there cultural, language, or accessibility considerations to keep in mind?
10. What specific outcomes should learners achieve by the end of the simulation?
11. How will the learning objectives align with organizational goals or patient care priorities?
12. Are the objectives measurable and actionable?
13. What organizational goals or initiatives does this simulation support?
14. Are there existing protocols, guidelines, or workflows that the simulation needs to incorporate?
15. What resources (time, budget, personnel) are available for designing and implementing this simulation?

16. Are there logistical constraints (e.g., scheduling, space, or equipment availability)?
17. What other training or simulations have been conducted recently, and how will this one build upon or complement them?
18. Who are the key stakeholders (e.g., department leaders, subject matter experts, educators)?
19. What input or expectations do stakeholders have for this simulation?
20. Are there any competing priorities or perspectives among stakeholders that need to be addressed?
21. What level of realism is necessary for the simulation to achieve its goals?
22. Can existing scenarios, materials, or resources be adapted, or will everything need to be developed from scratch?
23. What potential barriers could impact the success of this simulation, and how can they be mitigated?
24. How will we measure the success of the simulation?
25. What key performance indicators (KPIs) or metrics will demonstrate that learning objectives have been met?
26. What data or feedback will be collected during and after the simulation to inform future iterations?
27. How will this simulation contribute to the broader curriculum or professional development framework?
28. What are the expected long-term outcomes for learners and the organization?
29. How will we ensure that the skills or knowledge gained during the simulation are retained and applied in practice?

Key Takeaways

1. The Analyze phase is essential for understanding learner needs, defining audiences, and setting objectives, forming the foundation for successful healthcare simulations.
2. Effective needs analysis combines qualitative and quantitative methods, such as interviews, observations, and performance data.

3. Understanding the demographics, roles, and learning preferences of participants ensures simulations are relevant and engaging.
4. Clear and measurable objectives guide the design and evaluation of simulations, aligning training efforts with both learner and organizational goals.
5. Aligning training with organizational goals maximizes the impact of simulations on clinical performance and patient outcomes.

Reflection

The Analyze phase is where the seeds of effective healthcare simulations are sown. By investing time and effort into understanding training needs, defining the learner population, and setting clear objectives, educators lay a strong foundation for success. This phase is not just about identifying gaps; it is about envisioning the possibilities for growth and improvement.

Reflecting on the Analyze phase, consider how its principles can transform your approach to simulation design. How can you better understand your learners and their needs? Are your objectives truly aligned with clinical and organizational goals? By embracing the Analyze phase, you ensure the relevance of your simulations and enhance their potential to drive meaningful change in healthcare practice.

References

Branch, R. M. (2009). *Instructional design: The ADDIE approach.* Springer Science & Business Media.

Gagné, R. M., Wager, W. W., Golas, K. C., & Keller, J. M. (2005). *Principles of instructional design* (5th ed.). Wadsworth/Thomson Learning.

Hodell, C. (2016). ISD: From the ground up: A concise introduction to instructional design (4th ed.). American Society for Training and Development.

Kirkpatrick, D. L., & Kirkpatrick, J. D. (2006). *Evaluating training programs: The four levels.* Berrett-Koehler Publishers.

Morrison, G. R., Ross, S. M., Kalman, H. K., & Kemp, J. E. (2013). *Designing effective instruction* (7th ed.). Wiley.

Rosen, M. A., Salas, E., Silvestri, S., Wu, T. S., & Lazzara, E. H. (2008). Promoting teamwork: An event-based approach to simulation-based teamwork training for emergency medicine residents. *Academic Emergency Medicine, 15*(11), 1190-1198.

Zigmont, J. J., Kappus, L. J., & Sudikoff, S. N. (2011). The 3D model of debriefing: Defusing, discovering, and deepening. *Seminars in Perinatology, 35*(2), 52-58.

"Education is the kindling of a flame, not the filling of a vessel."
— Socrates

Chapter 3
Designing the Curriculum

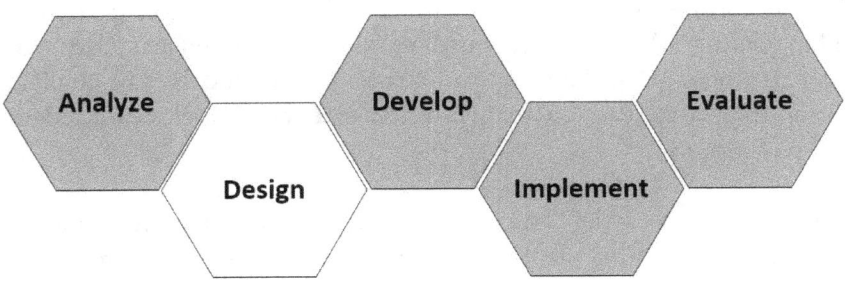

Designing the curriculum for healthcare simulation is where the creative vision comes to life. It's the phase where the insights gathered during analysis are transformed into a structured, engaging, and purposeful learning journey. Imagine constructing a bridge: every plank and beam must align with the overarching goal of guiding learners from where they are now to where they need to be. A well-designed simulation curriculum does precisely this—it connects learners' needs with the practical application of skills in a safe, controlled environment.

In this chapter, we'll explore the art and science of curriculum design. From building a framework that maps learning objectives to specific scenarios to incorporating learning theories that resonate with adult learners, we'll explore how to create impactful, evidence-based simulations. Additionally, we'll examine how to structure scenarios that mirror real-world clinical challenges and develop assessments that measure success with precision.

Building the Framework

A healthcare simulation curriculum must begin with a strong foundation. This foundation is built by aligning learning objectives with simulation scenarios that address the gaps identified during the Analyze phase. A curriculum without a clear framework is like a puzzle missing critical pieces—it may look promising at first glance but fails to deliver when tested.

Mapping Learning Objectives to Simulation Scenarios

Learning objectives are the north star of any simulation curriculum. They define what learners need to achieve and ensure that every scenario, activity, and debrief contributes to these goals. The challenge lies in translating these objectives into authentic and relevant scenarios for participants.

For example, consider a scenario aimed at improving communication in emergency trauma teams. The learning objectives might include:

1. Demonstrating clear and concise verbal communication.
2. Collaborating effectively under high-pressure conditions.
3. Prioritizing tasks based on the patient's immediate needs.

To meet these objectives, you might design a simulation involving a multidisciplinary response to a simulated motor vehicle accident. Learners could navigate challenges like role confusion, time constraints, and escalating patient instability. This scenario directly reflects the learning objectives, ensuring that the skills developed during the simulation translate seamlessly into real-world practice.

Sequencing Simulations for Impact

A thoughtfully sequenced curriculum ensures learners build their skills progressively. Start with simpler scenarios to establish foundational competencies and gradually introduce more complex challenges. This scaffolding approach helps learners gain confidence before tackling advanced tasks.

For instance, you might begin with basic newborn assessments in a neonatal care curriculum. Once learners demonstrate proficiency, they progress to more demanding scenarios, such as stabilizing a critically ill neonate or managing a neonatal resuscitation.

Incorporating Learning Theories

Your curriculum must be grounded in educational theories, particularly those suited for adult learners, to create meaningful learning experiences. These theories provide a roadmap for designing simulations that teach skills and inspire reflection and deeper understanding.

Applying Adult Learning Principles

Adult learners are distinct in their approach to education—they are practical, self-directed, and motivated by relevance. Malcolm Knowles' adult learning theory highlights several principles that resonate in healthcare simulation:

1. **Relevance:**

    Learners need to see the connection between what they're learning and their professional roles. A simulation that mirrors their daily challenges, such as managing sepsis in an ICU, will hold their attention far better than abstract content.

2. **Experience:**

Adults bring a wealth of prior knowledge to the table. Simulations that acknowledge and build on this experience foster a sense of competence and engagement.

3. **Problem-Solving:**

Adults learn best when faced with realistic problems. Scenarios that require critical thinking, such as triaging multiple patients in an emergency, challenge learners to think on their feet.

Experiential Learning in Action

Kolb's experiential learning theory emphasizes the importance of hands-on experiences in education. Healthcare simulations naturally align with this approach by allowing learners to:

1. Engage in a **concrete experience** during the simulation.
2. Reflect on their actions through structured debriefing (**reflective observation**).
3. Develop broader principles or strategies (**abstract conceptualization**) during the debrief.
4. Apply their new understanding to future scenarios (**active experimentation**).

For example, a simulation on patient handovers might highlight communication gaps. During debriefing, learners analyze their performance, identify areas for improvement, and brainstorm strategies for future handovers, completing Kolb's experiential cycle.

Scenario Planning

Designing a realistic and impactful scenario is both an art and a science. Scenarios are the heart of simulation-based learning, offering participants a safe space to practice, make mistakes, and grow.

Structuring Realistic and Evidence-Based Scenarios

A compelling scenario starts with a clear purpose. Every element—from the clinical context to the patient's symptoms—must support the learning objectives. The following components are essential:

- **Clinical Context:** To set the stage, define the environment (e.g., ICU, emergency room).
- **Learner Roles:** Specify roles for participants, such as team leader, bedside nurse, or respiratory therapist.
- **Patient Details:** Craft a patient history and current presentation that feel authentic.
- **Critical Events:** Include triggers that require learner action, such as a sudden decline in the patient's condition.
- **Desired Outcomes:** Define what success looks like, ensuring it aligns with the learning objectives.

For instance, a simulation on managing a patient with sepsis might start with subtle signs, such as a mild fever and elevated heart rate. If learners don't act quickly, the scenario escalates to septic shock, highlighting the importance of early intervention.

Balancing Realism and Practicality

While high-fidelity mannequins and advanced technology can enhance realism, they're not always necessary. The focus should be on creating a believable narrative, even with limited resources. For example, a well-written role-play scenario with detailed scripts can be as impactful as a high-tech simulation.

Assessment and Evaluation Strategies

Assessment and evaluation are essential components of the simulation design process. They serve as the bridge between the learning objectives established during the Analyze phase and the measurable outcomes of the simulation experience. Thoughtful assessment strategies ensure that simulations not only meet their intended goals but also provide learners with actionable feedback to enhance their clinical practice. Moreover, evaluations allow facilitators to identify areas of strength and improvement for future simulation iterations.

Designing Rubrics for Performance Assessment

Rubrics are invaluable tools for assessing learner performance in healthcare simulations. They provide a standardized method of evaluation, ensuring consistency and fairness while also aligning with the learning objectives. A well-constructed rubric does more than just evaluate performance—it serves as a guide for learners, clarifying expectations and helping them understand the key criteria for success.

Key Elements of Effective Rubrics

- **Alignment with Objectives:** Every criterion in the rubric must directly correspond to a specific learning objective. This alignment ensures that the assessment focuses on the intended outcomes rather than extraneous factors.
- **Clear, Specific Language:** Avoid vague terms like "good" or "poor," which can lead to inconsistent evaluations. Instead, use descriptors that clearly define the level of performance. For instance:
- **Excellent CPR Quality:** Maintains a depth of 5–6 cm and a rate of 100–120 compressions per minute consistently.
- **Needs Improvement in CPR Quality:** Depth and rate are frequently incorrect or inconsistent.
- **Multiple Domains:** Healthcare simulation assessments often involve three key domains:
- **Cognitive (Knowledge):** Understanding clinical guidelines or protocols.
- **Psychomotor (Skills):** Execution of physical tasks like performing chest compressions or administering medication.
- **Affective (Attitudes):** Demonstration of teamwork, empathy, or professionalism.

Example Rubric for a Cardiac Arrest Simulation

Criterion	Excellent	Competent	Needs Improvement
CPR Quality	Maintains correct depth	Occasional lapses in depth or rate	Frequently incorrect depth and rate

Criterion	Excellent	Competent	Needs Improvement
	and rate consistently		
Medication Administration	Administers correct dosage and timing every time	Minor timing or dosage errors	Frequent timing or dosage errors
Team Communication	Clear, concise, and inclusive of all team members	Adequate communication with occasional lapses	Communication is unclear or ineffective

This rubric provides clear, actionable feedback while aligning with the learning objectives of the simulation.

Formative and Summative Assessment

Assessment is not a one-time event. Effective evaluation strategies include formative and summative methods to provide comprehensive insights into learner performance.

Formative Evaluation

Formative evaluations are conducted during the simulation and focus on immediate feedback. This type of evaluation helps learners correct errors and refine their performance in real-time. Key elements include:

- **Facilitator Guidance:** Facilitators can pause the simulation briefly to address critical errors or offer coaching.
- **Observation Checklists:** Facilitators use checklists to monitor learner performance and provide targeted feedback.
- **Peer Feedback:** Learners can observe each other and offer constructive critiques during or after the simulation.

Example: In a neonatal resuscitation simulation, a facilitator might provide real-time feedback on hand positioning during chest compressions, allowing the learner to make immediate adjustments.

Summative Evaluation

Summative evaluations assess overall performance at the end of the simulation, measuring whether learners achieved the stated objectives. These evaluations are typically more formal and may include:

- **Facilitator Assessments:** Based on rubrics or checklists.
- **Self-Assessments:** Learners reflect on their own performance, identifying strengths and areas for improvement.
- **Knowledge Checks:** Quizzes or written tests can assess learners' understanding of protocols or guidelines.
- **Team Evaluations:** When simulations involve group dynamics, evaluate the team's overall effectiveness in meeting objectives.

Example: In a simulation focused on sepsis management, summative evaluation might involve a post-simulation quiz testing learners' knowledge of the sepsis protocol and a rubric-based assessment of their clinical actions during the scenario.

Advanced Evaluation Strategies

Debriefing as Part of Evaluation

Debriefing is an integral part of simulation-based learning and serves as both an evaluation and learning tool. During debriefing:

- Facilitators guide learners in reflecting on their actions and decisions.
- Key learning points are highlighted, reinforcing successes and addressing errors.
- Learners are encouraged to think critically about how they would apply their insights in real-world practice.

Performance Metrics and Data Collection

Incorporating technology into simulations allows for objective performance metrics. For instance:

- **Mannequin Data:** High-fidelity mannequins can record the depth and rate of chest compressions during CPR.
- **Video Analysis:** Recordings of the simulation can be reviewed to analyze team communication and decision-making.
- **Electronic Scoring Systems:** Automated systems can provide real-time scoring based on predefined criteria.

Longitudinal Assessment

Consider tracking learners' progress over time for simulations included in a broader curriculum. This method enables educators to evaluate the simulation's long-term effects and its incorporation into clinical practice.

The Role of Feedback in Assessment

Feedback is one of the most powerful tools in education. In simulations, it bridges the gap between performance and improvement:

- **Timeliness:** Immediate feedback during or after the simulation is more effective than delayed feedback.
- **Constructive Approach:** Focus on specific actions and behaviors rather than generalized praise or criticism.
- **Actionable Insights:** Provide clear recommendations for improvement and reinforce positive behaviors.

Example: Instead of saying, "Your communication needs work," a facilitator might say, "Next time, try summarizing your instructions to ensure everyone on the team understands their roles."

Bringing It All Together

Assessment and evaluation strategies ensure that simulations are more than just immersive experiences; they become measurable, impactful educational interventions. By designing rubrics, employing formative and summative evaluations, and providing actionable feedback, facilitators can help learners achieve their full potential while continuously refining the simulation. The goal is to assess and foster growth, ensuring that every simulation improves patient care and clinical outcomes.

Design Phase:
Questions to Ask

1. What are the specific skills, knowledge, or attitudes learners should gain from this simulation?
2. Are the objectives clear, measurable, and aligned with the outcomes identified during the analysis phase?
3. How will the learning objectives address the identified performance gaps or organizational goals?
4. Who are the learners, and what is their current level of knowledge and experience?
5. How can the simulation be designed to effectively engage the learners, considering their background and learning preferences?
6. Are there any specific accommodation or adjustments needed for the target audience?
7. What clinical situation or context best supports the learning objectives?
8. Is the scenario realistic and reflective of the learners' real-world challenges?
9. How will you structure the scenario? What roles, patient details, and triggers will you include?
10. What resources or tools (e.g., mannequins, technology, props) are necessary to create the scenario?
11. What teaching methods will be used? (e.g., experiential learning, role-play, case studies)
12. How will adult learning principles (e.g., relevance, problem-solving) be incorporated into the simulation?
13. What strategies will you use to foster critical thinking, teamwork, and decision-making skills?
14. How will learners be assessed during and after the simulation? What metrics or benchmarks will define success?
15. What assessment tools will you use? (e.g., checklists, rubrics, self-assessments)
16. How will feedback be provided to learners, and when? (e.g., during debriefing, post-simulation)
17. What logistical considerations (e.g., space, time, budget) must be factored into the design?
18. Can existing materials or resources be adapted, or will new ones need to be developed?
19. How will facilitators be trained to deliver the simulation effectively?

20. How will you measure the simulation's effectiveness in achieving its objectives?
21. What data will you collect to inform future iterations of the simulation?
22. How will the design allow for iterative improvements based on learner performance and feedback?

Detailed Role of Stakeholders in the Design Phase

The Design phase of the ADDIE model transforms the insights gathered during the Analysis phase into actionable plans for healthcare simulation. This phase focuses on developing structured learning objectives, scenario outlines, and assessment methods. Stakeholder involvement is essential during this phase to ensure that the design aligns with identified needs, professional standards, and organizational goals. Each stakeholder contributes expertise and perspective, making the final design both practical and impactful.

<u>Key Stakeholders and Their Roles</u>

Stakeholder	Role in Design Phase	Contributions
Educators	Shape learning objectives and instructional strategies to align with standards and needs.	- Define measurable objectives. - Propose teaching methods. - Align scenarios with curriculum goals.
Facilitators	Provide practical input on the feasibility and flow of scenarios.	- Suggest modifications for realism. - Advise on pacing and sequence. - Recommend debriefing strategies.
Administrators	Ensure design adheres to budget, resources, and organizational goals.	- Approve resources.

		- Align simulations with organizational initiatives. - Facilitate interdisciplinary collaboration.
Subject Matter Experts (SMEs)	Validate clinical accuracy and relevance of scenario content and objectives.	- Validate clinical details. - Suggest critical decision points. - Align design with evidence-based guidelines.
Learners	Offer feedback to ensure relevance, realism, and engagement.	- Provide feedback on draft scenarios. - Highlight preferred learning styles. - Identify engagement barriers.

Collaborative Effort for Comprehensive Design

The design process benefits from the collaboration of all stakeholders, ensuring that the simulation achieves its intended outcomes:

- **Educators** focus on pedagogy and curriculum alignment.
- **Facilitators** contribute practical insights to enhance realism and engagement.
- **Administrators** ensure feasibility within resource constraints.
- **SMEs** validate clinical accuracy and relevance.
- **Learners** ensure the design remains learner-centered and practical.

By working together, stakeholders ensure that the simulation design is not only feasible but also aligned with educational and organizational goals.

In the Design phase, stakeholders play vital roles in creating structured, learner-centered simulation plans that address identified needs and align with professional standards. Their combined expertise ensures that scenarios are realistic, engaging, and effective in achieving learning objectives. By fostering collaboration among educators, facilitators, administrators, SMEs, and learners, the Design phase creates a blueprint for impactful healthcare simulations.

The Design Phase: Inputs and Outputs

The Design phase of the ADDIE model translates the findings from the Analysis phase into a concrete instructional plan. This phase involves defining learning objectives, planning the training structure, and selecting methods, tools, and materials to be developed. The Design phase ensures that the curriculum aligns with learner needs and organizational goals, providing a detailed blueprint for the Development phase.

Inputs to the Design Phase

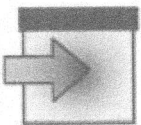

Inputs are the resources, findings, and deliverables from the Analysis phase that inform the planning and structuring of the training program.

Analysis Report
- Key findings from the Analysis phase, including identified gaps, learner profiles, and organizational goals.

    Example: The report highlights a need for ICU nurses to improve crisis communication and prioritization during emergencies.

Learning Needs and Objectives
- Initial high-level learning objectives derived from the Analysis phase.

    Example: Objectives like "recognize early signs of sepsis" or "demonstrate closed-loop communication during team scenarios."

Target Audience Profile

- Detailed demographics and learning preferences of the participants.

  Example: A mix of novice and experienced nurses, requiring tailored scenarios that address diverse skill levels.

Resource Inventory
- A list of available tools, technology, and materials, as well as any constraints such as budget or time.

  Example: Low-fidelity mannequins and a limited number of facilitators for a hospital training program.

Organizational Goals and Standards
- The training must align with broader goals, such as improving patient safety, reducing errors, or meeting accreditation standards.

  Example: Reducing medication errors by 20% within six months.

Outputs of the Design Phase

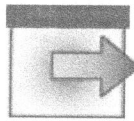
The outputs of the Design phase are the instructional plans, tools, and frameworks that guide the Development phase. These outputs ensure that the curriculum is structured, engaging, and aligned with the identified goals and objectives.

Detailed Learning Objectives
- Specific, measurable, achievable, relevant, and time-bound (SMART) objectives.

  Example: "By the end of the simulation, participants will correctly perform CPR within AHA guidelines for compression depth and rate."

Scenario Plans
- Detailed descriptions of simulation scenarios, including roles, events, and flow.

- *Example:* A trauma team scenario where participants must stabilize a patient with multiple injuries, manage a deteriorating airway, and communicate effectively.

Assessment Tools
- Rubrics, observation checklists, or scoring sheets to evaluate learner performance against objectives.

  Example: A rubric measuring technical skills, decision-making, and teamwork during a cardiac arrest simulation.

Instructional Strategies
- Chosen methods for delivering content, such as:
    - Case-based learning
    - Role-playing
    - High-fidelity simulations

  Example: Incorporating role-play to simulate nurse-family communication in a pediatric ICU scenario.

Pre-Simulation Materials
- Resources to prepare learners, such as:
    - Clinical guidelines
    - Case studies
    - Orientation videos

  Example: A video briefing on sepsis protocols and common challenges in early recognition.

Facilitator Guides
- Step-by-step instructions for facilitators, including scenario cues, timing, and debriefing questions.

  Example: A guide instructing facilitators to introduce a critical patient deterioration event at the midpoint of a simulation.

Storyboards or Flowcharts

- Visual representations of the sequence and flow of the scenarios.

    Example: A flowchart illustrating the progression of a neonatal resuscitation scenario, including branching options based on participant actions.

Evaluation Plan
- A framework for formative and summative assessments to measure success.

    Example: Formative evaluations during simulations and a post-training summative assessment via a knowledge test and performance review.

Design Phase	
Inputs	**Outputs (Deliverables)**
☐ Defined Learning Needs ☐ Target Audience Profile ☐ Learning Objectives ☐ Scope of Training ☐ Data-driven Insights ☐ Constraints & Assumptions ☐ Analysis Report	☐ Detailed Learning Objectives ☐ Scenario Plans ☐ Assessment Tools ☐ Instructional Strategies ☐ Pre-simulation Materials ☐ Facilitator Guides ☐ Storyboards/flowcharts ☐ Evaluation Plan

How Inputs Lead to Outputs

The Design phase uses inputs from the Analysis phase to create structured and actionable outputs. For example:

Input: Analysis reveals that novice nurses struggle with prioritizing tasks in emergencies.

Output: A scenario is designed where participants must prioritize interventions for a patient in septic shock, with measurable objectives like "correctly identify the three most critical interventions within 10 minutes."

By transforming raw data and needs into a detailed instructional plan, the Design phase ensures the curriculum is purposeful and effective.

The Design phase is the strategic backbone of the ADDIE model. It bridges the gap between identifying learning needs (inputs) and creating the materials and experiences (outputs) that address those needs. The Design phase lays the groundwork for a structured, engaging, and impactful training program by clearly defining objectives, developing scenarios, and planning assessments. This phase ensures that the training aligns with organizational goals and prepares learners for success in their real-world roles.

Key Takeaways

1. Designing a curriculum involves mapping learning objectives to scenarios, ensuring alignment and purpose.
2. Adult learning principles and experiential learning theories provide a strong foundation for engagement and retention.
3. Scenarios should balance realism with practical constraints while addressing specific learning objectives.
4. Effective rubrics and evaluations ensure learners achieve their goals and provide actionable feedback for improvement.

Reflection

As you reflect on the design process, consider:

1. **Alignment:** Do your scenarios and assessments align with the learning objectives?
2. **Engagement:** Are you incorporating principles that resonate with adult learners?
3. **Realism:** Have you struck the right balance between scenario complexity and feasibility?

4. **Feedback:** Are your assessment strategies robust and actionable?

Designing a curriculum is where vision becomes reality. By thoughtfully crafting scenarios, incorporating sound theories, and building robust assessments, you create simulations that not only educate but also transform how healthcare professionals approach patient care.

References

Branch, R. M. (2009). *Instructional design: The ADDIE approach.* Springer Science & Business Media.

Gagné, R. M., Wager, W. W., Golas, K. C., & Keller, J. M. (2005). *Principles of instructional design* (5th ed.). Wadsworth/Thomson Learning.

Hodell, C. (2016). ISD: From the ground up: A concise introduction to instructional design (4th ed.). American Society for Training and Development.

Jeffries, P. R. (2012). Simulation in nursing education: From conceptualization to evaluation. *National League for Nursing.*

Kolb, D. A. (1984). *Experiential learning: Experience as the source of learning and development.* Prentice Hall.

Knowles, M. S. (1980). *The modern practice of adult education: From pedagogy to andragogy.* Cambridge Books.

Morrison, G. R., Ross, S. M., Kalman, H. K., & Kemp, J. E. (2013). *Designing effective instruction* (7th ed.). Wiley.

Rosen, M. A., Salas, E., Silvestri, S., Wu, T. S., & Lazzara, E. H. (2008). Promoting teamwork: An event-based approach to simulation-based teamwork training for emergency medicine residents. *Academic Emergency Medicine, 15*(11), 1190-1198.

Zigmont, J. J., Kappus, L. J., & Sudikoff, S. N. (2011). The 3D model of debriefing: Defusing, discovering, and deepening. *Seminars in Perinatology, 35*(2), 52-58.

Chapter 4
Development

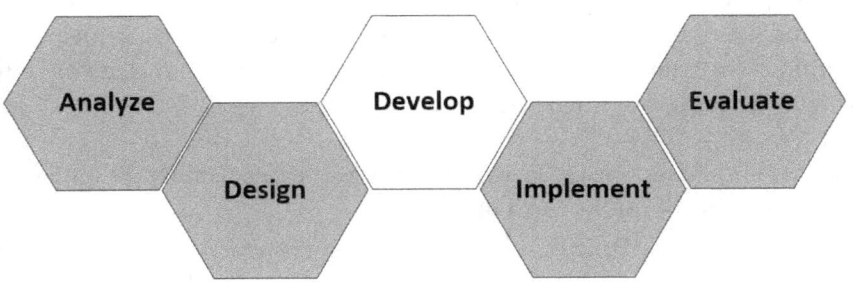

The Development Phase of the ADDIE model is where the vision crafted in the Design Phase begins to take shape. It's where plans become reality, creativity meets practicality, and every detail comes together to create an impactful and engaging simulation. Think of this phase as building a stage for a carefully choreographed performance. Every script, equipment, and environmental element must be precisely prepared to ensure the simulation runs smoothly.

This chapter will explore the intricate process of crafting content, preparing resources, and pilot testing simulations to refine them for optimal effectiveness. The goal of the Development Phase is not just to produce materials but to ensure that they are cohesive, aligned with learning objectives, and capable of delivering a transformative educational experience.

Creating Content

The heart of any simulation lies in its content. This includes the detailed scripts that guide the scenario, the case studies that frame the learning experience, and the facilitator guides that ensure consistency across sessions. Content creation is a meticulous process that requires attention to detail and a clear understanding of the learning objectives.

Crafting Detailed Scripts
Simulation scripts are much more than simple instructions; they are dynamic roadmaps that outline the simulation flow. A well-crafted script provides structure while leaving room for flexibility, allowing learners to explore and make decisions within the scenario.

Imagine a cardiac arrest scenario: The script doesn't just describe a patient collapsing; it provides a minute-by-minute breakdown of events, the patient's physiological responses, and the cues facilitators should use to guide learners. It might detail how a delay in administering epinephrine could result in worsening vital signs or how effective teamwork might stabilize the patient.

Scripts should anticipate learner actions and offer facilitators guidance on how to respond. For instance:
- **Trigger Points:** Include moments when the facilitator introduces changes, such as a sudden drop in blood pressure.
- **Learner Variability:** Prepare for different performance levels, ensuring the scenario can adapt to novices or advanced participants.

These scripts ensure that simulations are engaging and effective in meeting their learning objectives.

Developing Case Studies
Case studies add depth to the simulation experience. They serve as pre-simulation preparation tools or post-simulation discussion prompts, encouraging learners to connect clinical scenarios to broader concepts.

For example, consider a sepsis management simulation: The case study might begin with a detailed description of a patient presenting mild symptoms, such as fever and increased heart rate. Learners could analyze this information before the simulation to formulate potential diagnoses and treatment plans, which they then implement during the scenario. Case studies help bridge the gap between theoretical knowledge and practical application.

Creating Facilitator Guides

Facilitators are the conductors of the simulation orchestra, ensuring that all elements harmonize to create a meaningful experience. A robust facilitator guide equips them with everything they need to manage the simulation effectively, from setup to debriefing.

Facilitator guides should include:
- **Pre-Briefing Script:** A clear, step-by-step guide to prepare participants for the scenario and ensure they understand the objectives and expectations.
- **Scenario Overview:** A concise scenario summary, including learning objectives and key events.
- **Facilitation Strategies:** Instructions for managing timing, introducing cues, and addressing common challenges.
- **Debriefing Framework:** Structured questions that prompt learners to reflect on their performance and explore how they might apply lessons in real-world settings.

Example Debriefing Question: "How did your communication within the team impact the outcome of this scenario? What could you improve next time?"

Facilitator guides are invaluable in maintaining the integrity and consistency of the simulation across multiple sessions or instructors.

Selecting and Preparing Resources

The resources used in a simulation—from high-tech mannequins to simple props—play a pivotal role in creating a realistic and engaging environment. The selection process requires balancing educational goals, logistical considerations, and budget constraints.

Choosing Simulation Equipment
The type of equipment chosen should align with the complexity and fidelity of the simulation. High-fidelity mannequins, for instance, can simulate realistic physiological responses, while low-fidelity tools may suffice for basic skill training.

Example: A trauma simulation may require a high-fidelity mannequin with programmable vital signs and bleeding control features, whereas a scenario on medication administration might only need a simple injection pad.

Selecting the right equipment involves answering questions like:
- What level of realism is necessary to achieve the learning objectives?
- What is the learners' experience level, and how does the equipment support their needs?
- Are there budgetary or logistical constraints that must be considered?

Incorporating Technology

Technology can significantly enhance the simulation experience, providing learners with immersive and interactive tools. Examples include:
- **Virtual Reality (VR):** This technology allows learners to practice in environments like disaster zones or operating rooms without physical constraints.
- **Simulated Monitors:** Displaying vital signs that respond to learner actions in real-time.
- **Video Recording Systems:** Capturing simulations for review during debriefing, allowing learners to observe their actions objectively.

Preparing the Environment

The physical setting of the simulation should replicate the real-world clinical environment as closely as possible. This includes:

- **Room Setup:** Arranging furniture, equipment, and supplies to mimic the clinical setting (e.g., a hospital room or surgical suite).
- **Environmental Cues:** Adding background sounds, such as monitor alarms or patient moans, to heighten realism.
- **Accessibility:** Ensuring the setup is inclusive for all learners, including those with disabilities.
-

Example: For a home healthcare simulation, the environment might include a living room setup with common household hazards like loose rugs, requiring learners to identify safety risks as part of the scenario.

Pilot Testing

Pilot testing is where the rubber meets the road. It's the opportunity to test the simulation with a small group of participants and make adjustments before the full implementation.

Why Pilot Testing Matters

Pilot testing ensures the simulation is functional, realistic, and aligned with learning objectives. It allows developers to:
- Identify and fix technical issues with equipment or software.
- Refine the scenario's flow, ensuring it runs smoothly and within the allotted time.
- Gather feedback from participants and facilitators to identify areas for improvement.

Steps in Pilot Testing

1. **Choose Test Participants:** Select individuals whose expertise mirrors the target audience..
2. **Run the Simulation:** Execute the scenario as designed, paying close attention to timing, equipment performance, and participant engagement.
3. **Collect Feedback:** Use surveys or focus groups to understand participants' experiences and identify any challenges.
4. **Make Adjustments:** Based on feedback, refine scripts, guides, or equipment settings.

Example Refinement: During a neonatal resuscitation simulation pilot test, learners struggle to locate necessary equipment due to unclear labeling. In response, the development team reorganizes and labels the equipment to improve usability.

Development Phase:
Questions to Ask

1. Are the simulation scripts clear, detailed, and aligned with the learning objectives?
2. Do the scripts account for variability in learner actions, allowing for flexibility and adaptability?
3. Are the patient scenarios realistic and evidence-based?
4. Have case studies or pre-simulation materials been developed to prepare learners effectively?
5. Are facilitator guides comprehensive, providing clear instructions on managing the simulation and conducting debriefings?
6. Have you included specific prompts or cues for facilitators to assist learners in navigating the scenario?
7. Do the materials address potential challenges learners might face during the simulation?
8. What level of fidelity is required for the simulation to achieve its objectives?
9. Are the chosen resources (e.g., mannequins, technology, props) appropriate for the learners' skill level and the complexity of the scenario?
10. Do the resources align with the available budget and logistical constraints?
11. Have all technical requirements (e.g., software, monitors, audio-visual equipment) been identified and tested?
12. Are the resources reusable or adaptable for future simulations?
13. Is the physical environment suitable for the simulation? Does it replicate the real-world clinical setting?
14. Have you ensured accessibility for learners with disabilities or unique needs?
15. Does the simulation environment reflect the context and setting of the scenario (e.g., hospital room, operating theater, patient home)?
16. Are environmental cues, such as sounds or visual elements, realistic and relevant?
17. Does the scenario include clear triggers or critical events that require learner intervention?

18. Have you planned for role assignments (e.g., team leader, observer) and ensured they align with the learning objectives?
19. Have you identified a small group of participants for pilot testing who resemble the target audience?
20. Have you planned how to collect feedback from pilot participants (e.g., surveys, focus groups)?
21. Are the facilitators adequately trained to deliver and evaluate the simulation during the pilot test?
22. Have you scheduled time to refine the simulation based on pilot test feedback?
23. Are there contingency plans for technical issues or unexpected challenges during pilot testing?
24. Does the simulation include mechanisms to capture data (e.g., video recordings, performance metrics) for analysis and feedback?
25. Are there clear criteria for determining the success of the pilot test?
26. Have you planned how to integrate learner and facilitator feedback into refinements?
27. Are the assessments (e.g., rubrics, checklists) clear and aligned with the learning objectives?
28. Have you tested the timing of the simulation to ensure it fits within the allocated session?
29. Are all materials, resources, and technology fully functional and ready for implementation?
30. Have you reviewed the simulation flow to identify and address any potential bottlenecks or ambiguities?
31. Have you conducted a final review with subject matter experts to confirm accuracy and relevance?
32. Do you have contingency plans in place for any unexpected issues during implementation?

Detailed Role of Stakeholders in the Development Phase

The Development phase in the ADDIE model is where the plans from the Design phase come to life. This stage involves creating and assembling instructional materials, tools, and resources needed for the simulation. Collaboration among stakeholders is critical to ensure that the outputs of this phase align with the objectives, are functional, and meet the learners' and organization's needs. Each stakeholder brings unique insights and expertise, contributing to the successful creation of high-quality simulations.

Key Stakeholders and Their Roles

Stakeholder	Role in Development Phase	Contributions
Educators	Ensure materials and tools align with pedagogical goals and learning objectives.	- Review draft materials. - Develop pre-simulation resources. - Validate instructional guides.
Facilitators	Test and refine simulations for practicality, realism, and learner engagement.	- Pilot test scenarios. - Suggest adjustments for flow and engagement. - Refine facilitator instructions.
Administrators	Oversee resource allocation and ensure compliance with budget and policies.	- Approve equipment and technology. - Manage logistics for materials. - Ensure alignment with policies.
Subject Matter Experts (SMEs)	Provide clinical expertise to validate accuracy and authenticity of content.	- Review scripts for accuracy. - Provide input on patient presentations. - Suggest evidence-based practices.
Learners	Offer feedback during pilot testing to improve clarity, realism, and usability.	- Test usability of materials. - Provide feedback on instructions. - Highlight confusing or unrealistic elements.

Collaborative Effort for Successful Development

The Development phase requires close collaboration among stakeholders to ensure that the materials and tools are:
- **Educator-Validated:** Aligned with curriculum goals and designed for effective learning.
- **Facilitator-Tested:** Practical, engaging, and reflective of real-world scenarios.
- **Administrator-Supported:** Backed by adequate resources and organizational approval.
- **SME-Endorsed:** Clinically accurate and relevant.
- **Learner-Reviewed:** User-friendly and suited to the learners' needs and experiences.

In the Development phase, stakeholders bring their expertise to ensure the quality and relevance of simulation materials. Educators validate the educational content, facilitators refine the practicality, administrators provide resources, SMEs ensure clinical accuracy, and learners offer critical feedback. By working together, these stakeholders ensure the creation of effective and impactful healthcare simulations.

The Development Phase: Inputs and Outputs

The Development phase of the ADDIE model is where the instructional plans from the Design phase are brought to life. This phase involves creating, assembling, and testing the materials, tools, and resources used during the Implementation phase. The success of this phase depends on the quality and accuracy of the inputs from the Design phase and the systematic creation of outputs that align with the instructional goals.

Inputs to the Development Phase

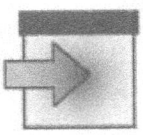

Inputs are the resources, plans, and data generated during the Design phase that inform the creation of instructional materials.

Scenario Plans and Design Documents
- Detailed descriptions of scenarios, including roles, events, flow, and objectives.

  Example: A trauma simulation scenario with a flowchart of critical events, such as a sudden drop in blood pressure or a cardiac arrest.

Learning Objectives
- Specific and measurable objectives that guide the creation of materials and assessments.

  Example: "Learners will perform CPR within AHA guidelines for rate and depth during the simulation."

Assessment Tools and Evaluation Frameworks
- Rubrics, checklists, or performance criteria for evaluating learner success.

  Example: An observation checklist for team communication and adherence to clinical protocols during a simulation.

Facilitator Guides
- Step-by-step instructions for facilitators, including scenario cues, timing, and debriefing prompts.

  Example: A guide instructing facilitators to trigger a simulated patient deterioration event 10 minutes into the scenario.

Pre-Simulation Materials
- Learner resources, such as case studies, instructional videos, or clinical guidelines, are designed to prepare participants.

  Example: A video on sepsis management protocols to be viewed before participating in a simulation.

Resource Inventory
- A list of available equipment, technology, and tools, as well as identified constraints.

Example: High-fidelity mannequins, VR systems, or low-fidelity props depending on the budget and scope.

Storyboards and Flowcharts
- Visual representations of scenario sequences and decision points.

Example: A storyboard for a neonatal resuscitation scenario showing the timeline of events and branching options based on participant actions.

Outputs of the Development Phase

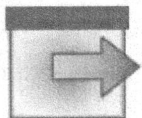

The outputs of the Development phase are the tangible materials, resources, and tools created for the training program. These outputs must align with the instructional goals and be ready for implementation.

Simulation Scenarios and Scripts
- Fully developed scenarios with detailed scripts for facilitators and standardized patients (if applicable).

Example: A cardiac arrest simulation script detailing patient vitals, facilitator cues, and expected learner actions.

Instructional Materials
- Learner resources, such as:
    - Pre-simulation briefings or handouts.
    - Case studies and reference guides.

Example: A clinical guideline booklet on managing sepsis and a pre-simulation quiz to assess baseline knowledge.

Assessment Tools
- Finalized rubrics, observation checklists, and scoring sheets for evaluating learner performance.

Example: A rubric measuring technical skills, decision-making, and teamwork during a trauma response simulation.

Facilitator Resources
- Detailed guides for facilitators, including:
    - Scenario cues and decision triggers.
    - Debriefing questions and evaluation instructions.

Example: A facilitator guide for an interdisciplinary team training simulation with critical thinking and communication prompts.

Simulation Environment Setup
- Creation of the physical or virtual environment where the simulation will occur

Example: A trauma bay setup with mannequins, monitors, and props like blood bags and surgical instruments.

Technology and Media Development
- Creation or integration of multimedia elements, such as:
    - Virtual reality (VR) scenarios.
    - Augmented reality (AR) overlays.
    - Videos and animations.

Example: A VR simulation where learners practice intubating a patient in a high-pressure environment.

Tested Materials
- All materials and resources were tested for functionality, usability, and alignment with objectives.

Example: Conducting a trial run of a sepsis management simulation to ensure timing and cues flow smoothly.

Revised and Finalized Content
- Updates made to materials based on pilot testing or stakeholder review feedback.

Example: Revising a scenario script after pilot testing reveals that learners need more time to make decisions during critical events.

Development Phase	
Inputs	**Outputs (Deliverables)**
☐ Detailed Learning Objectives ☐ Scenario Plans ☐ Assessment Tools ☐ Instructional Strategies ☐ Pre-simulation Materials ☐ Facilitator Guides ☐ Storyboards/flowcharts ☐ Evaluation Plan	☐ Simulation Scenarios & Scripts ☐ Instructional Materials ☐ Assessment Tools ☐ Facilitator Resources ☐ Simulation Environment Setup ☐ Technology & Media Development ☐ Tested Materials ☐ Revised & Finalized Content

How Inputs Lead to Outputs

The Development phase transforms the abstract plans and frameworks of the Design phase into actionable, tangible materials. For instance:

Input: A scenario plan outlines a simulation where learners must manage a patient in septic shock.

Output: A fully developed scenario script with detailed cues for facilitators, patient vitals, and a checklist to assess learner performance.

The systematic use of inputs ensures that outputs align with the instructional goals and are ready for seamless implementation.

The Development phase is the creative and production hub of the ADDIE model, where the instructional vision becomes reality. By leveraging detailed plans and resources from the Design phase, this phase produces high-quality materials and environments that facilitate effective learning. Outputs from the Development phase must be tested, refined, and aligned with objectives to ensure they are ready for successful delivery in the Implementation phase.

Key Takeaways

1. Content creation in the Development Phase includes crafting scripts, case studies, and facilitator guides that align with learning objectives.
2. Selecting appropriate resources, from high-fidelity mannequins to realistic environments, enhances the simulation's impact.
3. Pilot testing is essential for identifying and addressing issues, ensuring the simulation is both effective and engaging.

Reflection

The Development Phase is where ideas transform into actionable tools. By embracing creativity, attention to detail, and iterative improvement, the Development Phase sets the stage for delivering simulations that prepare learners to excel in real-world clinical environments. It's a meticulous process, but one that ultimately transforms vision into reality

References

Branch, R. M. (2009). *Instructional design: The ADDIE approach*. Springer Science & Business Media.

Fanning, R. M., & Gaba, D. M. (2007). The role of debriefing in simulation-based learning. *Simulation in Healthcare, 2*(2), 115-125.

Gaba, D. M. (2004). The future vision of simulation in healthcare. *Quality and Safety in Health Care, 13*(Suppl 1), i2-i10.

Gagné, R. M., Wager, W. W., Golas, K. C., & Keller, J. M. (2005). *Principles of instructional design* (5th ed.). Wadsworth/Thomson Learning.

Hodell, C. (2016). ISD: From the ground up: A concise introduction to instructional design (4th ed.). American Society for Training and Development.

Jeffries, P. R. (2012). Simulation in nursing education: From conceptualization to evaluation. *National League for Nursing*.

Morrison, G. R., Ross, S. M., Kalman, H. K., & Kemp, J. E. (2013). *Designing effective instruction* (7th ed.). Wiley.

Rosen, M. A., Salas, E., Wu, T. S., Silvestri, S., & Lazzara, E. H. (2008). Promoting teamwork: An event-based approach to simulation-based teamwork training for emergency medicine residents. *Academic Emergency Medicine, 15*(11), 1190-1198.

Zigmont, J. J., Kappus, L. J., & Sudikoff, S. N. (2011). The 3D model of debriefing: Defusing, discovering, and deepening. *Seminars in Perinatology, 35*(2), 52-58.

KEITH A. BEAULIEU

"Learning never exhausts the mind."
— Leonardo da Vinci

Chapter 5
Implementation in Healthcare Simulation

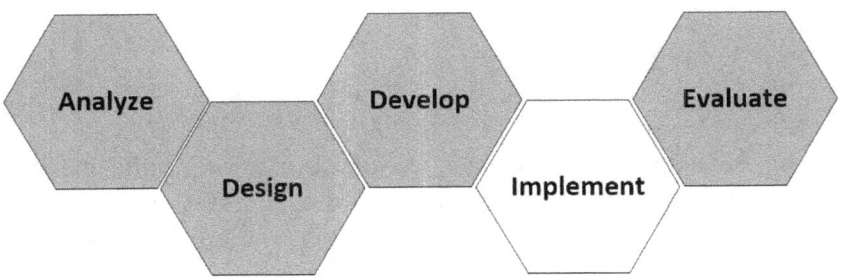

The Implementation Phase is the pivotal moment when all the preparation, creativity, and effort invested in the earlier phases come to fruition. It is where the vision takes center stage, facilitators step into their roles, and learners engage in scenarios designed to challenge, educate, and inspire. The success of this phase depends on more than just running the simulation—it requires meticulous planning, effective facilitation, and a readiness to adapt to the unexpected.

Think of implementation as conducting a symphony. Every element—the facilitators, the participants, the environment, and the resources—must work in harmony. However, even with precise preparation, unexpected notes may arise, and the conductor must guide the ensemble back on track. In healthcare simulation, facilitators take on this role, orchestrating a seamless learning experience while ensuring flexibility to address challenges. This chapter delves into launching the curriculum, mastering the art of facilitation, and navigating obstacles to create impactful simulations.

Launching the Curriculum

Before the first simulation session begins, much of the behind-the-scenes work ensures that everything runs smoothly. This phase involves coordinating logistics, setting up environments, and preparing facilitators and participants to achieve the intended outcomes.

Managing Logistics and Scheduling

Logistics can make or break a simulation program. The devil is in the details, and overlooking even minor elements can disrupt an otherwise well-designed simulation. From scheduling sessions to setting up the physical environment, careful planning ensures that participants can focus entirely on learning.

Key Steps in Managing Logistics:

- **Scheduling Sessions:** Align simulation dates and times with the availability of learners, facilitators, and resources. For large groups, consider staggered sessions or smaller cohorts to maximize participation and engagement.

    Example: A hospital implementing a new code blue protocol might schedule multiple sessions over a week to train all shifts.

- **Preparing the Physical Environment:** The simulation space should replicate the clinical environment as closely as possible. Every detail, from bed placement to equipment setup, contributes to the realism of the scenario.

    Example: For a labor and delivery simulation, ensure the environment includes birthing beds, fetal monitors, and relevant emergency equipment.

- **Testing Equipment:** Before the session, verify that all equipment, technology, and audiovisual tools are functioning. A malfunction during the session can disrupt the flow and diminish the learning experience.

Preparing Facilitators and Participants

Preparation is the foundation of a successful simulation. Facilitators must be confident in guiding the session, while participants need to understand the objectives and what to expect.

Facilitator Preparation:
- Conduct a pre-implementation meeting to walk facilitators through the scenario, learning objectives, and their roles.
- Provide facilitator guides with detailed instructions, cues, and debriefing prompts.
- Practice mock simulations to build familiarity with the equipment and scenario flow.
- Anticipate potential questions or challenges and prepare strategies to address them.

Participant Preparation:
- Offer pre-simulation materials, such as clinical guidelines, case studies, or orientation videos, to help participants arrive informed and ready to engage.
- Brief participants on the simulation's purpose and structure, emphasizing that the goal is learning, not evaluation.

Example: "This simulation is a safe space to practice critical skills. Mistakes are expected and part of the learning process."

Address common anxieties by reassuring participants that performance during the simulation is not tied to punitive consequences but is an opportunity to grow.

Effective Facilitation

Facilitators are the linchpin of a successful simulation. Their ability to guide learners, create a psychologically safe environment, and foster critical thinking can make the difference between a good simulation and a transformative one.

Techniques for Guiding Learners

Facilitation is a dynamic process that requires balancing structure with flexibility. Facilitators must know when to intervene, when to step back, and how to steer discussions toward meaningful learning.

- **Establish Psychological Safety:** From the outset, facilitators should create an atmosphere where learners feel comfortable taking risks and making mistakes.

  Example: Start with an icebreaker or a light discussion to ease tensions and build rapport with participants.

- **Encourage Learner Autonomy:** Allow learners to take the lead in decision-making and problem-solving, stepping in only when necessary to keep the scenario on track.

  Example Prompt: "What's your next step in managing this patient's declining oxygen saturation?"

- **Adapt to the Group's Needs:** Tailor facilitation techniques to the learners' experience level. For novices, provide more prompts and cues; for advanced learners, challenge their critical thinking and teamwork skills.

Debriefing as the Heart of Facilitation

Debriefing is often regarded as the most crucial part of a simulation. It transforms the experience into actionable insights, giving learners the chance to reflect on their performance, connect it to clinical principles, and plan for improvement.

Debriefing Framework:
- **Defusing:** Start by addressing participants' immediate reactions to the simulation. This helps them process emotions and focus on learning

Example Question: "What was your initial reaction to the patient's sudden decline?"

- **Discovering:** Facilitate a discussion about the actions taken during the simulation. Encourage participants to identify strengths, areas for improvement, and the rationale behind their decisions.

  Example Question: "What went well during the team's response, and where do you see opportunities for improvement?"

- **Deepening:** Connect the discussion to broader clinical knowledge and practice. This is the moment to reinforce key takeaways and inspire learners to apply them in real-world settings.

- **Example Prompt:** "How can these communication strategies help prevent errors in your clinical practice?"

Handling Challenges

No matter how meticulously the simulation is planned, unexpected challenges are inevitable. The key to successful implementation is anticipating potential issues and adapting.

Common Challenges and Solutions

- **Technical Failures:** Equipment malfunctions, such as mannequins freezing or monitors failing, can disrupt the session.
    - **Solution:** Have backup plans, such as manual data sheets or verbal cues, to keep the simulation moving.

- **Learner Anxiety:** Some participants may feel intimidated by the simulation environment.
    - **Solution:** Normalize mistakes as part of the learning process and remind participants of the session's supportive nature.

- **Time Constraints:** Scenarios running longer than planned can leave little time for debriefing.
    - **Solution:** Prioritize critical moments during debriefing and schedule follow-up discussions if necessary.
- **Group Dynamics:** Unequal participation or conflicts among team members can hinder the simulation.
    - **Solution:** Intervene diplomatically, encouraging all participants to contribute while maintaining group harmony.

Turning Challenges into Opportunities

Challenges often provide valuable insights into future improvements. After each session, gather feedback from participants and facilitators to identify areas of strength and opportunities for refinement.

Feedback Questions:
- What aspects of the simulation were most helpful to your learning?
- Were there any moments that felt unrealistic or confusing?
- What could be improved for future sessions?

By viewing challenges as opportunities for growth, facilitators can continuously enhance the simulation experience.

Implementation Phase
Questions to Ask

1. Are the simulation sessions scheduled at times that accommodate all participants, including facilitators and learners?
2. Do the simulation spaces reflect the intended clinical or educational environment?
3. Is all the necessary equipment (e.g., mannequins, technology, props) available and functional?
4. Have backup resources been identified in case of equipment failures?

5. Have facilitators been adequately briefed on their roles, the learning objectives, and the simulation flow?
6. Do facilitators feel confident managing the technical and educational aspects of the simulation?
7. Are there clear guides or scripts available for facilitators to reference during the session?
8. Have learners received pre-simulation materials, such as case studies, procedural guidelines, or orientation videos?
9. Do learners understand the objectives of the simulation and their roles within it?
10. Have learners been informed about the session's structure, including debriefing and assessment components?
11. How will you establish psychological safety for learners, ensuring they feel comfortable making mistakes and learning from them?
12. Have ground rules been communicated, such as the confidentiality of discussions and the focus on learning rather than evaluation?
13. Are the scenarios realistic and appropriately challenging for the learners' experience level?
14. How will facilitators balance guidance with allowing learners to problem-solve independently?
15. Are there contingency plans for unexpected learner actions that deviate from the scenario?
16. What is the protocol if technical issues arise during the simulation?
17. How will facilitators handle scenarios that take more or less time than expected?
18. Can facilitators address group dynamics, such as dominant or disengaged participants?
19. Is there a clear plan for debriefing sessions, including defusing emotions, discovering learning points, and deepening understanding?
20. How will facilitators ensure that all learners have an opportunity to reflect and contribute during debriefing?
21. What specific questions or prompts will facilitators guide reflection and discussion?
22. How will immediate feedback be provided during or after the simulation to address critical errors?
23. Are there strategies to ensure feedback is constructive, actionable, and focused on performance improvement?

24. Are assessment tools (e.g., checklists, rubrics) aligned with the learning objectives and being used consistently?
25. How will facilitator observations and learner self-assessments be collected and analyzed?
26. What performance metrics (e.g., response times, communication effectiveness) will be recorded during the session?
27. Are there plans to collect learner feedback on the simulation's realism, relevance, and impact?
28. How will facilitators debrief to discuss what worked and what could be improved?
29. Are there mechanisms to capture lessons learned and refine future sessions based on feedback?
30. Did the simulation achieve its intended learning objectives?
31. Are there opportunities to enhance the simulation's realism, flow, or impact in future iterations?

Detailed Role of Stakeholders in the Implementation Phase

The Implementation phase of the ADDIE model is where the simulation is delivered to learners. This phase involves setting up the environment, executing the simulation scenarios, and guiding learners through the experience. Effective implementation requires stakeholder collaboration to ensure the simulation runs smoothly, achieves its objectives, and creates a supportive learning environment. Each stakeholder brings a unique perspective and set of responsibilities that contribute to the success of the implementation.

<u>Key Stakeholders and Their Roles</u>

Stakeholder	Role in Implementation Phase	Contributions
Educators	Oversee simulation delivery and ensure alignment with learning objectives.	- Facilitate pre-simulation briefings. - Monitor learner engagement. - Provide immediate feedback during or after the session.

Facilitators	Guide learners through scenarios, manage pacing, and ensure smooth flow.	- Manage pacing and triggers in scenarios. - Observe performance and behaviors. - Conduct debriefing sessions.
Administrators	Coordinate logistics, resources, and scheduling to support implementation.	- Schedule sessions and ensure availability of resources. - Address logistical or technical issues. - Support cross-department coordination.
Subject Matter Experts (SMEs)	Validate real-time accuracy of clinical scenarios and provide expert insights.	- Validate clinical accuracy during sessions. - Address learner questions about clinical practices. - Provide targeted feedback.
Learners	Engage actively in simulations and provide feedback on the experience.	- Demonstrate skills and knowledge in scenarios. - Reflect during debriefing. - Share feedback on realism and relevance.

Collaborative Effort for Successful Implementation

During the Implementation phase, stakeholders work together to ensure that simulations achieve their intended objectives:

- **Educators** provide guidance and feedback to help learners connect the simulation experience with real-world applications.
- **Facilitators** manage the scenario's flow and ensure that learners stay engaged and focused.
- **Administrators** coordinate the logistical elements, ensuring the simulation environment is prepared and resources are available.
- **SMEs** ensure clinical accuracy and offer expert insights.

- **Learners** actively engage and provide feedback to enhance the experience.

The Implementation phase is a collaborative effort that brings simulation to life. Each stakeholder contributes to its success, from educators and facilitators guiding the session to administrators ensuring logistical support and SMEs maintaining clinical relevance. Learners benefit from this teamwork, gaining practical experience in a supportive, realistic environment. By clearly defining roles and fostering collaboration, the Implementation phase maximizes the impact of healthcare simulations.

The Implementation Phase: Inputs and Outputs

The Implementation phase is where the instructional materials, simulations, and plans created during the Development phase are delivered to learners. This phase ensures that the curriculum is effectively executed, learners are prepared, and facilitators are equipped to deliver the training. A successful implementation phase depends on using high-quality inputs and producing impactful outputs that align with the instructional objectives.

Inputs to the Implementation Phase

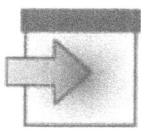

This phase's inputs include all the preparation, materials, and resources developed in the earlier phases, ensuring readiness for effective delivery.

Simulation Scenarios and Scripts

- Detailed scenarios with clear instructions for facilitators and participants.

    Example: A trauma simulation script where facilitators introduce patient deterioration cues at specific times.

Facilitator Guides

- Comprehensive guides outlining facilitator roles, scenario flow, and debriefing instructions.

  Example: A guide for a sepsis management simulation, including when and how to provide cues for escalation events.

Instructional Materials
- Learner-focused resources, such as pre-simulation handouts, guidelines, and orientation materials.

  Example: A clinical protocol guide provided to learners before the simulation.

Assessment Tools
- Rubrics, checklists, and scoring sheets to evaluate learner performance during the simulation.

  Example: A rubric assessing technical skills, teamwork, and decision-making in a cardiac arrest scenario.

Simulation Environment Setup
- A physical or virtual environment that mimics the clinical setting, including necessary equipment and technology.

  Example: An ICU setup with mannequins, monitors, and props like syringes and ventilators.

Technology and Equipment
- Fully functional tools, such as high-fidelity mannequins, VR systems, or augmented reality overlays.

  Example: A virtual reality system enabling learners to practice surgical techniques in a risk-free environment.

Learner and Facilitator Preparation
- Pre-simulation activities to orient learners and facilitators, ensuring clarity on objectives and roles.

Example: A pre-briefing session where facilitators review the learning objectives and learners discuss their expectations.

Scheduling and Logistics Plan

- A detailed schedule for simulation sessions, including assigned roles, timing, and location.

Example: A week-long training schedule with staggered nursing and medical staff sessions.

Outputs of the Implementation Phase

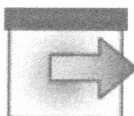

The outputs of the Implementation phase reflect the successful execution of the training, including learner engagement, data collection, and immediate feedback.

Delivered Simulation Sessions

- Execution of the planned simulations with active learner participation.

Example: A high-fidelity trauma simulation where learners respond to critical events in real time.

Learner Engagement and Participation

- Active involvement of learners in the training is demonstrated through teamwork, decision-making, and problem-solving.

Example: A team of nurses collaboratively managing patient care during a pediatric emergency simulation.

Facilitator Performance

- Effective guidance from facilitators, including scenario management and delivery of feedback.

Example: A facilitator ensures smooth scenario progression and uses structured prompts during the debriefing session.

Performance Data Collection

- Data was gathered during the simulation for later analysis and evaluation.

  Example: Metrics like CPR compression quality or response time to patient deterioration events recorded during the session.

Formative Feedback for Learners
- Immediate, constructive feedback provided during or after the simulation.

  Example: Facilitators offering insights into team communication gaps during the debrief.

Debriefing Sessions
- Structured discussions where learners reflect on their performance, identify strengths and explore areas for improvement.

  Example: A post-simulation debrief exploring how a delayed response to a critical event impacted patient outcomes.

Identified Challenges or Gaps
- Document any issues encountered during the simulation, such as technical difficulties or unclear instructions.

  Example: Facilitators noted that learners struggled with identifying key patient symptoms, suggesting a need for pre-simulation reinforcement.

Feedback from Participants
- Insights from learners and facilitators about the simulation's realism, relevance, and effectiveness.

  Example: Learners providing feedback that the scenario felt highly realistic but that additional time for decision-making would enhance the experience.

Implementation Phase	
Inputs	**Outputs (Deliverables)**
☐ Simulation Scenarios & Scripts ☐ Instructional Materials ☐ Assessment Tools ☐ Facilitator Resources ☐ Simulation Environment Setup ☐ Technology & Media Development ☐ Tested Materials ☐ Revised & Finalized Content	☐ Delivered Simulation Sessions ☐ Learner Engagement & Participation ☐ Facilitator Performance ☐ Performance Data Collection ☐ Formative Feedback for Learners ☐ Debriefing Sessions ☐ Identified Challenges or Gaps ☐ Feedback from Participants

How Inputs Lead to Outputs

The Implementation phase transforms the well-prepared inputs into actionable learning experiences. For instance:

Input: A facilitator guide details specific events, such as when to simulate a patient's oxygen saturation drop.

Output: Facilitators introduce these events during the simulation, engaging learners in critical decision-making and problem-solving.
The quality of the inputs directly impacts the effectiveness of the outputs, ensuring that learners achieve the intended objectives.

The Implementation phase is where preparation meets action. It combines all the earlier phases' materials, environments, and plans to deliver immersive and meaningful training experiences. By leveraging robust inputs and focusing on learner engagement, formative feedback, and data collection, this phase ensures that the curriculum is delivered effectively, setting the stage for evaluation and continuous improvement.

Key Takeaways

1. Effective implementation requires meticulous logistical planning, including scheduling, setup, and equipment testing.
2. Preparing facilitators and participants ensures everyone is confident and ready to engage.
3. Facilitation techniques, such as establishing psychological safety and conducting thoughtful debriefs, create a supportive and impactful learning environment.
4. Challenges are inevitable, but a proactive mindset and adaptability can turn obstacles into learning opportunities.

Reflection

The Implementation Phase is the culmination of the ADDIE process. By approaching this phase with flexibility, creativity, and a learner-centered mindset, you can create simulation experiences that leave a lasting impact, equipping healthcare professionals to excel in their roles and improve patient outcomes.

References

Branch, R. M. (2009). *Instructional design: The ADDIE approach.* Springer Science & Business Media.

Fanning, R. M., & Gaba, D. M. (2007). The role of debriefing in simulation-based learning. *Simulation in Healthcare, 2*(2), 115–125. https://doi.org/10.1097/SIH.0b013e3180315539

Gaba, D. M. (2004). The future vision of simulation in healthcare. *Quality and Safety in Health Care, 13*(Suppl 1), i2–i10. https://doi.org/10.1136/qshc.2004.009878

Hodell, C. (2016). ISD: From the ground up: A concise introduction to instructional design (4th ed.). American Society for Training and Development.

Jeffries, P. R. (2012). Simulation in nursing education: From conceptualization to evaluation. *National League for Nursing.*

Kolb, D. A. (1984). *Experiential learning: Experience as the source of learning and development.* Prentice Hall.

Rosen, M. A., Hunt, E. A., Pronovost, P. J., Federowicz, M. A., & Weaver, S. J. (2012). In situ simulation in continuing education for the healthcare professions: A systematic review. *Journal of*

Continuing Education in the Health Professions, 32(4), 243–254. https://doi.org/10.1002/chp.21152

Zigmont, J. J., Kappus, L. J., & Sudikoff, S. N. (2011). The 3D model of debriefing: Defusing, discovering, and deepening. *Seminars in Perinatology, 35*(2), 52–58. https://doi.org/10.1053/j.semperi.2011.01.003

Chapter 6
Evaluation and Feedback

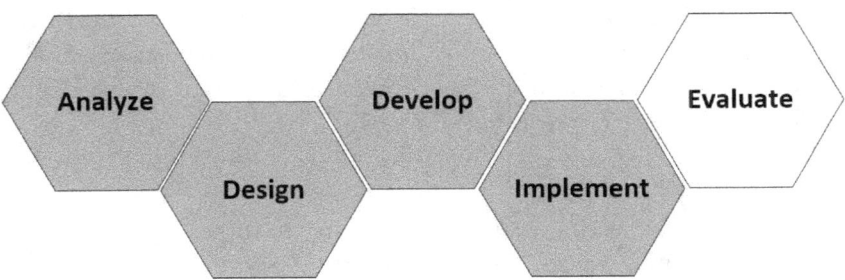

The Evaluation Phase is the cornerstone of the ADDIE model's promise of continuous improvement. This phase is not merely about closing the loop on a training cycle; it's about opening the door to new opportunities for refinement and growth. In healthcare simulation, where the stakes are high, and outcomes can have life-altering implications, the role of evaluation extends beyond checking boxes. The mechanism transforms a good simulation into a great one and, ultimately, a transformative learning experience.

Imagine evaluation as the lens that brings clarity to your work. Through this lens, you uncover what worked, what didn't, and what needs adjustment. Quantitative and qualitative feedback becomes the compass guiding your future efforts. Evaluation ensures that every element of the simulation, from the design of the scenarios to the facilitation techniques, evolves in response to the needs of learners and the ever-changing healthcare landscape.

In this chapter, we will explore the role of evaluation in the ADDIE process, delve into the tools and methods that make it effective, and discuss how to use feedback to iterate on and enhance the simulation curriculum.

Role of Evaluation in ADDIE

Evaluation serves two vital purposes in the ADDIE model: **ensuring continuous improvement** and **providing accountability.** It allows instructional designers and facilitators to determine whether a simulation has met its intended objectives and, more importantly, how it can be refined to serve learners and the organization better.

Ensuring Continuous Improvement

The value of evaluation lies in its iterative nature. In healthcare simulation, no design is ever truly "finished." Clinical practices evolve, technologies advance, and learner needs shift. Evaluation provides the feedback necessary to adapt and improve.

Example:

Consider a simulation designed to improve team communication during emergency trauma care. In its first iteration, feedback might reveal that learners felt unprepared for the pace of the scenario. Based on this insight, you might adjust the pre-simulation briefing to include a focused discussion on managing high-pressure situations. In the next iteration, you might evaluate whether this change improved learner confidence and performance.

Accountability

The evaluation also ensures that the simulation delivers measurable value. Whether administrators, educators, or learners, stakeholders want evidence that the training achieves its goals. A robust evaluation process provides data to support the investment in simulation.

Example:

A hospital invests in simulations to reduce medication errors. Through evaluation, facilitators collect data on error rates during the simulation, track learner improvement over time, and demonstrate a corresponding decline in real-world medication errors post-training. This evidence strengthens the case for continued simulation-based education.

Tools and Methods for Assessment

Effective evaluation requires the right tools and methods. These should align with the simulation's learning objectives and provide actionable insights. A combination of **formative** and **summative assessments** is essential to capture a complete picture of the simulation's impact.

Formative and Summative Assessments

- **Formative Assessments:** These are conducted during the simulation or immediately after each session to provide real-time feedback. They help facilitators address issues as they arise and allow learners to make immediate adjustments.

- *Example:* A facilitator observes that a learner hesitates to initiate chest compressions during a neonatal resuscitation simulation. The facilitator pauses the simulation to provide guidance, allowing the learner to correct their approach in the moment.

- Tools: Checklists, observation forms, and immediate feedback discussions.

Summative Assessments occur after the simulation program and evaluate whether the learning objectives were achieved. Summative assessments provide a more comprehensive picture of overall effectiveness.

- *Example:* A summative evaluation might include a post-simulation test where learners demonstrate their ability to identify and manage septic shock in a standardized scenario.

- Tools: Rubrics, post-simulation quizzes, and performance analytics.

Gathering Feedback from Learners and Facilitators

Feedback is the heart of the Evaluation Phase. It provides a window into the learner's experience, highlights the simulation's strengths, and identifies areas for improvement.

Learner Feedback:

- **Surveys:** Structured surveys can capture data on various simulation aspects, such as realism, difficulty, and overall satisfaction.

  Example Question: "How confident do you feel applying the skills practiced in this simulation to a real clinical setting?"

- **Self-Assessments:** Encourage learners to reflect on their performance and identify personal areas for growth.

  Example Question: "What is one skill you feel you improved on during this simulation?"

- **Focus Groups:** Provide a space for in-depth discussions where learners can share their experiences and suggestions.

Facilitator Feedback:

- **Post-Simulation Debriefs:** Facilitators can reflect on what went well, where learners struggled, and what adjustments might enhance the experience.

  Example Question: "Did the scenario progress as expected, or were there unexpected learner actions that required on-the-spot adjustments?"

- **Facilitator Surveys:** These can evaluate the usability of the facilitator guides, the functionality of the equipment, and the simulation's overall flow.

Quantitative and Qualitative Methods

Evaluation is most effective when it combines quantitative data, which provides measurable results, and qualitative insights, adding depth and context.

Quantitative Tools:
- Rubrics that measure specific skills, such as correct medication administration or adherence to clinical protocols.
- Pre- and post-simulation tests to evaluate knowledge retention.
- Performance data from high-fidelity mannequins, such as CPR depth or response time.

Qualitative Tools:
- Open-ended survey questions that allow learners to articulate their thoughts and feelings.
- Video reviews of the simulation, which facilitators can analyze to identify nuanced behaviors, such as nonverbal communication or leadership dynamics.

Iterating on the Curriculum

The insights gained during the Evaluation Phase are only as valuable as the actions they inspire. Iteration is using evaluation outcomes to refine the simulation curriculum, ensuring it becomes more effective with each cycle.

Refining the Design Based on Evaluation Outcomes
- **Analyzing Data:** Identify trends in learner performance and feedback to pinpoint areas that need adjustment.

  Example: If learners struggle with closed-loop communication, consider adding a pre-simulation workshop or incorporating specific prompts during the scenario.

- **Addressing Gaps:** Use evaluation data to determine whether any learning objectives were not fully met and modify the scenario accordingly.

Example: If a sepsis management simulation reveals that learners are slow to recognize signs of septic shock, consider including a pre-simulation review of diagnostic criteria.

- **Incorporating Feedback:** Act on suggestions from learners and facilitators to improve realism, flow, and overall engagement.

Example: Facilitators suggest adding a time-out feature to address learner confusion during high-pressure scenarios.

Examples of Iterative Improvements

Scenario Refinement: A trauma simulation originally included a complex series of injuries that overwhelmed learners. After evaluation, the injuries were simplified, and a second session was added to increase their complexity gradually.

Enhanced Resources: Learners reported difficulty understanding the simulation objectives, leading to the creation of detailed pre-simulation briefings.

Improved Debriefing Practices: Facilitators noted inconsistent debriefs across sessions, prompting the adoption of a structured framework, such as the "Defuse, Discover, Deepen" model.

Evaluation Phase:
Questions to Ask
1. Did the simulation meet the intended learning objectives?
2. Could learners demonstrate the skills, knowledge, or attitudes outlined in the objectives?
3. Were the scenarios realistic and relevant to the learners' clinical roles and responsibilities?
4. Did learners feel prepared to apply their knowledge to real-world situations?
5. How did learners perceive the simulation? Was it engaging and challenging?
6. What aspects of the simulation did learners find most beneficial?

7. Were there any elements of the simulation that learners found confusing or unnecessary?
8. Did learners feel supported by facilitators during the session?
9. Were pre-simulation materials (e.g., case studies, guidelines) helpful in preparing learners?
10. Were facilitators confident and comfortable delivering the simulation?
11. Did the facilitator guide provide sufficient instructions and support?
12. Were there any points in the simulation where facilitators struggled to manage timing, learner actions, or technical elements?
13. What improvements do facilitators suggest for the scenario or debriefing process?
14. Were the evaluation tools (e.g., rubrics, checklists) effective in measuring learner performance?
15. Did formative assessments provide timely and actionable feedback during the simulation?
16. Were summative assessments aligned with the learning objectives?
17. How did learners respond to feedback provided during debriefing?
18. Did all equipment and technology function correctly during the simulation?
19. Were there any technical issues that disrupted the learning experience?
20. Was the physical environment conducive to achieving the simulation's goals?
21. Were logistical elements, such as scheduling and resource allocation, well-managed?
22. What specific suggestions did learners provide for improving the simulation?
23. Did facilitators offer insights into areas that could enhance scenario realism or flow?
24. Are there any patterns or common themes in the feedback collected?
25. What changes could make the simulation more effective or engaging in the future?
26. Are there gaps in the curriculum that need to be addressed in future simulations?

27. How can feedback from this evaluation cycle be incorporated into the next iteration of the simulation?
28. What new trends or advancements in healthcare should be considered for future updates to the curriculum?
29. Did the simulation support organizational goals, such as improving patient safety or enhancing teamwork?
30. How can the data from this evaluation be used to demonstrate the value of the simulation to stakeholders?
31. What long-term impact do you anticipate from this simulation on learner performance or patient outcomes?

Detailed Role of Stakeholders in the Evaluation Phase

The Evaluation phase of the ADDIE model is critical for determining the success of a healthcare simulation program. It involves assessing whether learning objectives were achieved, identifying areas for improvement, and measuring the overall effectiveness of the simulation. This phase relies heavily on input from various stakeholders, each contributing unique perspectives to ensure a comprehensive evaluation. Collaboration among stakeholders ensures the evaluation process is thorough, actionable, and aligned with the program's goals.

Key Stakeholders and Their Roles

Stakeholder	Role in Evaluation Phase	Contributions
Educators	Analyze learner outcomes to determine if objectives were met and identify gaps for improvement.	- Analyze performance data. - Recommend changes to learning objectives. - Evaluate assessment alignment with standards.
Facilitators	Provide observational insights into learner performance and the effectiveness of scenario execution.	- Highlight effective and ineffective scenario elements. - Offer feedback on debriefing processes.

		- Identify areas for refinement.
Administrators	Evaluate program impact, including ROI and alignment with organizational priorities.	- Review program outcomes and resource allocation. - Approve funding for refinements. - Facilitate cross-departmental evaluations.
Subject Matter Experts (SMEs)	Ensure the clinical accuracy and relevance of evaluation tools and scenarios.	- Review learner adherence to clinical benchmarks. - Validate evaluation tools and metrics. - Recommend updates to clinical scenarios.
Learners	Reflect on their experience, providing feedback to improve the simulation process.	- Share challenges and suggestions during post-simulation discussions. - Complete surveys and self-assessments. - Reflect on skill application.

Collaborative Effort for Comprehensive Evaluation

A successful evaluation requires the active participation of all stakeholders to ensure that all aspects of the simulation are assessed:

- **Educators** focus on the alignment of learner outcomes with instructional goals.
- **Facilitators** provide observational feedback on the flow and execution of scenarios.
- **Administrators** assess the program's overall impact and ROI.
- **SMEs** validate the clinical relevance and accuracy of the evaluation process.
- **Learners** offer firsthand insights into the simulation's effectiveness and areas for improvement.

This collaborative approach ensures that the evaluation process is robust, actionable, and targeted toward continuous improvement.

The Evaluation phase is a team effort that measures the effectiveness of the simulation and identifies areas for refinement. Educators analyze learner outcomes, facilitators provide observational insights, administrators review program impact, SMEs ensure clinical accuracy, and learners offer valuable feedback. By leveraging the expertise and perspectives of all stakeholders, the evaluation phase drives continuous improvement and maximizes the impact of healthcare simulations.

The Evaluation Phase: Inputs and Outputs

The Evaluation phase of the ADDIE model serves as the quality control step, assessing the effectiveness of the training program and identifying areas for improvement. This phase collects and analyzes data to determine if the learning objectives were achieved, how well the simulation was delivered and what changes might enhance future iterations. Evaluation ensures accountability, drives continuous improvement, and closes the loop in the instructional design process.

Inputs to the Evaluation Phase

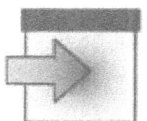

The evaluation phase's inputs come from data, tools, and feedback gathered during the previous phases, especially Implementation. These inputs provide the raw material for assessing the program's effectiveness.

Learning Objectives
- Specific and measurable objectives defined during the Design phase.

    Example: "Demonstrate proper closed-loop communication during a trauma resuscitation scenario."

Assessment Tools
- Rubrics, observation checklists, and scoring sheets developed during the Design and Development phases.

    Example: A checklist tracking learner adherence to clinical protocols during the simulation.

Performance Data

- Metrics gathered during the Implementation phase, such as:
  - Time-to-intervention.
  - Accuracy of skills performed.
  - Decision-making quality.

  Example: Data showing that 80% of participants completed CPR correctly within the specified time frame.

Learner Feedback
- Post-simulation surveys, self-assessments, and focus group discussions reflecting learner experiences.

  Example: Learners report that the simulation was realistic but needed clearer pre-simulation instructions.

Facilitator Feedback
- Observations and insights from facilitators about the scenario flow, learner engagement, and potential improvements.

  Example: Facilitators note that participants struggled with understanding role assignments, suggesting the need for clearer instructions.

Simulation Observations
- Notes and recordings from facilitators or evaluators about how learners performed during the simulation.

  Example: Observers document that learners consistently missed early signs of patient deterioration.

Organizational Goals and Metrics
- Broader outcomes the training aims to influence, such as reduced error rates or improved teamwork.

  Example: Tracking whether a simulation-based sepsis training program led to a decrease in response times in real clinical settings.

Outputs of the Evaluation Phase

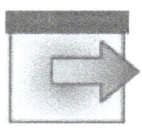 The outputs of the Evaluation phase are the actionable results and insights that determine the program's success and guide future iterations. These outputs inform both the immediate refinement of the program and its long-term effectiveness.

Evaluation Report
- A comprehensive document summarizing the findings, including:
    - Whether learning objectives were met.
    - Strengths and weaknesses of the program.
    - Recommendations for improvement.

Example: A report showing that while learners mastered technical skills, they needed additional practice in team communication.

Performance Metrics
- Quantitative and qualitative data showing how well learners performed relative to the objectives.

Example: 90% of learners successfully identified signs of sepsis, but only 60% escalated care within the required timeframe.

Participant Feedback Summary
- An analysis of learner feedback highlighting areas of satisfaction and concern.

Example: Participants found the scenarios realistic but requested more time for debriefing sessions.

Facilitator Feedback Summary
- Insights from facilitators about scenario flow, resources, and learner engagement.

Example: Facilitators suggest adding more dynamic events to challenge advanced learners.

Recommendations for Refinement
- Specific suggestions for improving the simulation curriculum.

    Example: Enhance pre-simulation materials to include a tutorial on using specific equipment.

Actionable Changes for Future Iterations
- Concrete updates to materials, scenarios, or delivery methods.

    Example: Modifying the scenario script to introduce clearer role assignments during the pre-briefing.

Organizational Impact Data
- Evidence showing how the training influenced real-world outcomes.

    Example: A hospital reports a 15% reduction in medication errors following a simulation-based safety training program.

Iterative Design Plan
- A roadmap for applying the evaluation results to improve the program in the next cycle.

    Example: A revised design plan incorporating additional scenarios to address gaps in clinical decision-making.

Evaluation Phase	
Inputs	**Outputs (Deliverables)**
☐ Learning Objectives ☐ Assessment Tools ☐ Performance Data ☐ Learner Feedback ☐ Facilitator Feedback ☐ Simulation Observations ☐ Organizational Goals & Metrics	☐ Evaluation Report ☐ Performance Metrics ☐ Participant Feedback Summary ☐ Facilitator's Feedback Summary ☐ Recommendations for Refinement

	☐ Actionable Changes for Future Interventions ☐ Organizational Impact Data ☐ Iterative Design Plan

How Inputs Lead to Outputs

The Evaluation phase processes the inputs gathered during the Implementation phase and transforms them into meaningful outputs. For example:

Input: Learner performance data shows delays in recognizing septic shock during the simulation.

Output: It is recommended that pre-simulation training be added on early warning signs of sepsis.

By analyzing inputs systematically, the Evaluation phase ensures that the outputs directly address learner needs and organizational goals.

The evaluation phase is crucial for ensuring the simulation program remains effective, relevant, and continuously improving. This phase produces actionable outputs such as evaluation reports, refinement recommendations, and measurable evidence of program impact by utilizing robust inputs like performance data and participant feedback. The insights gained validate the program's success and foster innovation and adaptation, ensuring the curriculum evolves to meet the changing demands of healthcare education.

Key Takeaways

1. Evaluation is essential for measuring success, ensuring accountability, and driving continuous improvement.
2. Formative and summative assessments provide immediate and long-term insights into the simulation's impact.
3. Gathering feedback from learners and facilitators enriches the evaluation process and highlights actionable areas for refinement.

4. Iterative improvements based on evaluation data ensure that the simulation curriculum evolves to meet the changing needs of learners and the healthcare environment.

Reflection

Evaluation is the catalyst for growth and innovation in healthcare simulation. Treating it as an ongoing process rather than a final step ensures that each simulation meets its objectives and continuously pushes the boundaries of what learners can achieve.

References

Branch, R. M. (2009). *Instructional design: The ADDIE approach*. Springer Science & Business Media.

Fanning, R. M., & Gaba, D. M. (2007). The role of debriefing in simulation-based learning. *Simulation in Healthcare, 2*(2), 115–125. https://doi.org/10.1097/SIH.0b013e3180315539

Gaba, D. M. (2004). The future vision of simulation in healthcare. *Quality and Safety in Health Care, 13*(Suppl 1), i2–i10. https://doi.org/10.1136/qshc.2004.009878

Hodell, C. (2016). *ISD: From the ground up: A concise introduction to instructional design* (4th ed.). American Society for Training and Development.

Jeffries, P. R. (2012). Simulation in nursing education: From conceptualization to evaluation. *National League for Nursing*.

Kirkpatrick, D. L., & Kirkpatrick, J. D. (2006). *Evaluating training programs: The four levels*. Berrett-Koehler Publishers.

Kolb, D. A. (1984). *Experiential learning: Experience as the source of learning and development*. Prentice Hall.

Morrison, G. R., Ross, S. M., Kalman, H. K., & Kemp, J. E. (2013). *Designing effective instruction* (7th ed.). Wiley.

Zigmont, J. J., Kappus, L. J., & Sudikoff, S. N. (2011). The 3D model of debriefing: Defusing, discovering, and deepening. *Seminars in Perinatology, 35*(2), 52–58. https://doi.org/10.1053/j.semperi.2011.01.003

"The capacity to learn is a gift; the ability to learn is a skill; the willingness to learn is a choice."
— Brian Herbert

Chapter 7
Resource Allocation Across Phases in the ADDIE Model

Resource allocation is the backbone of any successful instructional design project, especially in healthcare simulation where precision, realism, and impact are critical. Each phase of the ADDIE model demands a unique blend of time, personnel, tools, and budget. Effective planning and allocation ensure that every phase is well-supported, fostering a seamless workflow that leads to meaningful learning experiences and measurable outcomes. This chapter dives into the specific resource needs for each phase, providing detailed guidance and healthcare-specific examples to illustrate how resources can be optimized.

1. Analyze Phase: Laying the Groundwork

The Analyze phase sets the foundation for the entire instructional design process. It identifies gaps, defines learning needs, and aligns training objectives with organizational goals. This phase requires deliberate planning and resource allocation to ensure comprehensive and actionable data collection and analysis.

Resource Needs

- **Time:** Moderate to significant, depending on the complexity of the training needs.
- **Personnel:**
  - **Educators and facilitators** to assess learner needs.
  - **Administrators** to provide organizational data and support.
  - **SMEs** to validate findings and guide the focus of the simulation.
- **Budget:** Minimal to moderate, especially if using external surveys or focus group facilitators.
- **Technology:** Data collection tools include surveys, performance dashboards, and feedback platforms.

Healthcare Example:
Imagine a hospital experiencing high rates of sepsis-related complications. The Analyze phase might include reviewing patient safety reports, conducting focus groups with frontline staff, and surveying knowledge gaps about sepsis protocols. This effort involves time from educators, data analysts, and clinical SMEs to identify precise areas for improvement.

2. Design Phase: Crafting the Blueprint

The Design phase transforms raw data from the Analyze phase into a structured plan. This stage is where learning objectives are defined, scenarios are outlined, and assessments are planned. The complexity of this phase often requires significant time and cross-disciplinary collaboration to ensure that designs align with learner needs and professional standards.

Resource Needs

- **Time:** Significant, as this phase involves iterative planning and multiple reviews.
- **Personnel:**
  - **Instructional designers** to map out learning objectives and activities.
  - **Facilitators** to ensure feasibility and realism in scenarios.

- - SMEs to validate clinical content.
- **Budget:** Moderate, especially if external consultation or advanced tools are needed.
- **Technology:** Storyboarding software, simulation scenario planning tools, and LMS platforms.

Healthcare Example:
Designing a trauma team communication simulation for an emergency department requires careful planning. Educators work with SMEs to outline key decision points, facilitators ensure the scenarios are logistically viable, and instructional designers align objectives with ACGME standards for teamwork and communication. This phase requires moderate financial investment in design tools and team collaboration.

3. Development Phase: Bringing the Plan to Life

The Development phase is the creative hub of the ADDIE model, where simulation materials, resources, and tools are created. This phase often demands the most significant resource allocation, as it involves content creation, pilot testing, and refining materials for optimal impact.

Resource Needs

- **Time:** High, as materials must be developed, tested, and refined.
- **Personnel:**
  - **Developers and designers** to create and assemble resources.
  - **Facilitators and SMEs** to test scenarios and provide feedback.
  - **Administrators** to coordinate logistics.
- **Budget:** Significant, particularly if high-fidelity mannequins, VR platforms, or custom software are involved.
- **Technology:** Simulation software, multimedia tools, and physical equipment like mannequins and medical devices.

Healthcare Example:
Creating a VR-based simulation for neonatal resuscitation training involves programming a realistic clinical environment, pilot testing with facilitators, and refining based on learner feedback. This phase often requires external vendors for technology development and substantial budget allocation for equipment and software licenses.

4. Implementation Phase: Delivering the Experience

The Implementation phase brings the simulation to learners, translating months of planning and development into actionable training experiences. This phase focuses on ensuring the simulation environment is ready, learners are prepared, and the scenarios are executed seamlessly.

Resource Needs

- **Time:** Moderate, depending on the number and frequency of simulation sessions.
- **Personnel:**
    - **Facilitators** to guide simulations and manage debriefing sessions.
    - **Technicians** to troubleshoot equipment and ensure smooth operation.
    - **Administrators** to manage scheduling and logistics.
- **Budget:** Moderate, covering costs for facilitator hours, equipment maintenance, and participant logistics.
- **Technology:** Fully operational simulation setups, audiovisual systems, and evaluation tools.

Healthcare Example:
Delivering a simulation on managing cardiac arrest requires skilled facilitators to guide learners through Advanced Cardiac Life Support (ACLS) protocols, technicians to maintain and operate mannequins, and administrators to ensure efficient scheduling. Time is allocated to both the simulation and subsequent debriefing to maximize learning outcomes.

5. Evaluation Phase: Measuring Success

The Evaluation phase ensures that the simulation has achieved its objectives and identifies opportunities for improvement. This phase involves analyzing learner performance data, gathering feedback, and refining materials for future iterations.

Resource Needs

- **Time:** Moderate, for data collection, analysis, and reporting.
- **Personnel:**
  - **Evaluators** to assess outcomes and identify gaps.
  - **Facilitators** to provide observational insights.
  - **SMEs** to validate the alignment of outcomes with clinical benchmarks.
- **Budget:** Minimal to moderate, depending on the sophistication of assessment tools.
- **Technology:** Assessment tools, data analytics platforms, and feedback collection systems.

Healthcare Example:
Evaluating a medication safety simulation might involve analyzing rubric data, reviewing learner feedback forms, and comparing pre- and post-simulation error rates. SMEs ensure evaluation tools are clinically valid, while administrators review ROI to support program sustainability.

Maximizing Resource Efficiency

Prioritize High-Impact Areas: Allocate more resources to phases directly influencing outcomes, such as Development and Evaluation.

Leverage Technology: Use tools like simulation software and learning management systems to streamline processes and reduce manual effort.

Collaborate Effectively: Engage stakeholders early to identify and plan for resource needs collaboratively.

Iterate and Improve: Use feedback and evaluation data to refine resource allocation for future projects.

Resource allocation is a critical aspect of implementing the ADDIE model in healthcare simulation. Programs can maximize efficiency and effectiveness by understanding the specific resource needs of each phase and tailoring strategies to meet those needs. Proper planning ensures that healthcare simulations achieve their educational objectives and create meaningful, lasting impacts on learner performance and patient care. Through thoughtful resource management, the ADDIE model becomes a powerful framework for driving excellence in healthcare education.

ADDIE Workflow vs. Effort

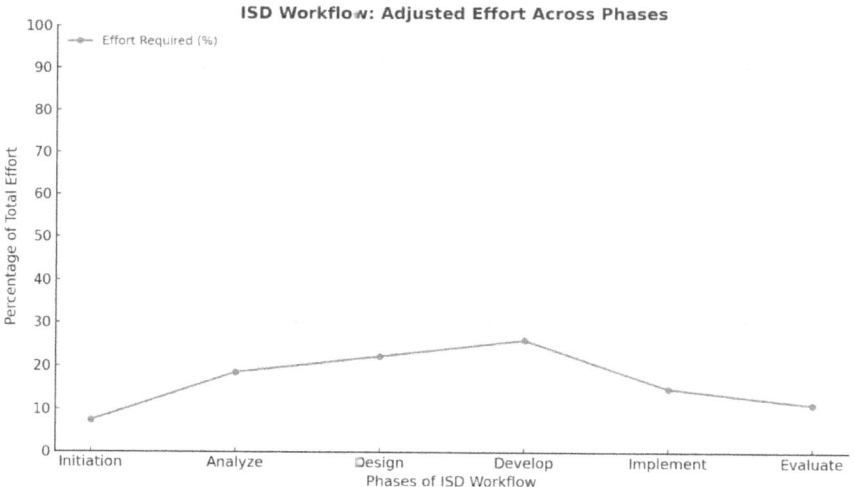

The graph illustrates the proportional effort required across the phases of the ISD workflow, adjusted to total 100%. Each phase represents a percentage of the total effort, emphasizing the following insights:

Effort Distribution:
- The **Design** and **Develop** phases require the highest effort, reflecting the complexity of creating instructional materials, simulation scenarios, and assessment tools.

- Moderate effort is needed during the **Analyze** phase to identify needs, define objectives, and align with organizational goals.
- The **Implement** phase requires slightly less effort, as it focuses on executing the prepared curriculum and gathering immediate feedback.
- **Initiation** and **Evaluate** require the least effort, as they are more about planning and assessment rather than intensive development.

Implications:
- Programs should allocate the majority of resources (time, personnel, and tools) to the Design and Develop phases for a high-quality output.
- Evaluation, though requiring less effort, is critical for ensuring continuous improvement and program effectiveness.

Purpose:
- This distribution highlights the importance of prioritizing effort where it has the greatest impact, ensuring that the instructional design process is efficient and effective.
- The graph provides a clear visual representation to guide resource allocation in ISD projects, particularly in environments like healthcare simulation where time and effort must be optimized.

Example:

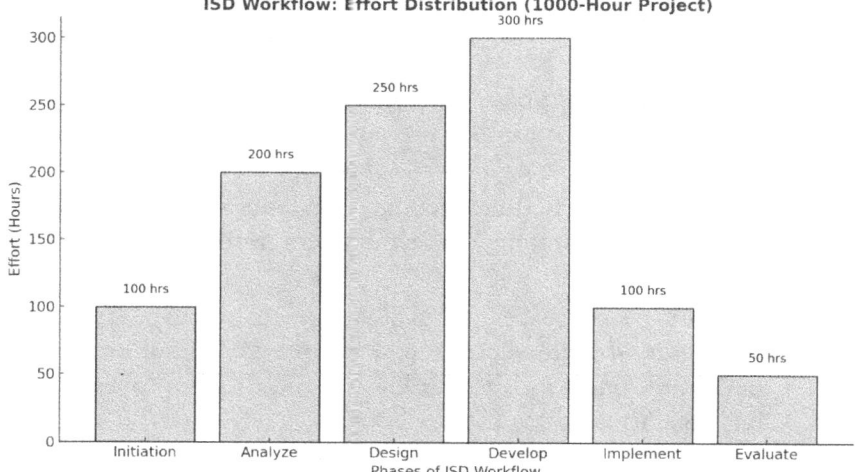

The graph above illustrates the distribution of effort across the phases of the ISD workflow for a sample 1,000-hour project. It highlights the hours allocated to each phase based on their adjusted percentage of total effort:

- **Initiation:** 100 hours
- **Analyze:** 200 hours
- **Design:** 250 hours
- **Develop:** 300 hours
- **Implement:** 100 hours
- **Evaluate:** 50 hours

This visualization emphasizes the need to focus resources on the Design and Develop phases, which require the most effort while maintaining proportional attention to the other phases to ensure project success.

Note: The ratio of time spent on the Implementation phase compared to the other phases combined is approximately 1:9, meaning the Implementation phase requires about 11% of the total time allocated to all other phases.

Key Takeaways

1. Resource Needs Vary Across Phases
   - Each phase of the ADDIE model—Analyze, Design, Develop, Implement, Evaluate—requires unique resource allocations in terms of time, personnel, budget, and technology.
   - Understanding these needs ensures that resources are distributed effectively to support each phase's goals.
2. Critical Phases Demand More Resources
   - The Development phase often demands the highest resource investment, involving content creation, pilot testing, and refinement.
   - The Evaluation phase, while less resource-intensive, plays a critical role in ensuring continuous improvement and alignment with objectives.
3. Stakeholder Collaboration is Essential
   - Engaging stakeholders like educators, facilitators, administrators, SMEs, and learners ensures comprehensive planning and effective resource use.
   - Collaborative input helps identify priorities and mitigate resource constraints.
4. Technology Amplifies Efficiency
   - Tools like simulation software, learning management systems, and analytics platforms streamline processes, saving time and reducing manual effort.
   - Leveraging technology can enhance outcomes while optimizing resource use.
5. Iterative Feedback Drives Improvement
   - Using feedback and evaluation results to adjust resource allocation ensures better outcomes in future projects.
   - Reallocation based on real-world results allows for more strategic planning and execution.

Reflection

Resource allocation is often an overlooked component of instructional design, yet it determines the success of every phase in the ADDIE model. Reflecting on the nuances of each phase reveals how critical proper planning is—not just for achieving objectives but for maintaining efficiency and stakeholder satisfaction.

In healthcare simulation, the stakes are particularly high. Misallocation of resources could lead to ineffective simulations, wasted budgets, or even reduced learner engagement. However, with thoughtful planning and collaboration, resource allocation becomes an enabler of impactful training.

- Consider these questions as you reflect on resource management in your own projects:
- Are you allocating sufficient resources to the phases that demand the most investment, such as Development?
- Have you engaged all stakeholders to ensure your resource planning accounts for diverse needs and perspectives?
- Are you leveraging technology to streamline processes and reduce costs?

By addressing these questions and applying the principles discussed in this chapter, you can transform resource management from a challenge into a strength, ensuring that your healthcare simulations are efficient, effective, and transformative.

Resources

Branch, R. M. (2009). *Instructional design: The ADDIE approach.* Springer Science & Business Media.

Gagné, R. M., Wager, W. W., Golas, K. C., & Keller, J. M. (2005). *Principles of instructional design* (5th ed.). Wadsworth/Thomson Learning.

Hodell, C. (2016). *ISD: From the ground up: A concise introduction to instructional design* (4th ed.). American Society for Training and Development.

Kirkpatrick, D. L., & Kirkpatrick, J. D. (2006). *Evaluating training programs: The four levels.* Berrett-Koehler Publishers.

Morrison, G. R., Ross, S. M. Kalman, H. K., & Kemp, J. E. (2013). *Designing effective instruction* (7th ed.). Wiley.

Rosen, M. A., Hunt, E. A., Pronovost, P. J., Federowicz, M. A., & Weaver, S. J. (2012). In situ simulation in continuing education for the healthcare professions: A systematic review. *Journal of Continuing Education in the Health Professions, 32*(4), 243–254. https://doi.org/10.1002/chp.21152

Svinicki, M. D., & McKeachie, W. J. (2014). *McKeachie's teaching tips: Strategies, research, and theory for college and university teachers* (14th ed.). Wadsworth Cengage Learning.

Zigmont, J. J., Kappus, L. J., & Sudikoff, S. N. (2011). The 3D model of debriefing: Defusing, discovering, and deepening. *Seminars in Perinatology, 35*(2), 52–58. https://doi.org/10.1053/j.semperi.2011.01.003

"**Learning is a treasure that will follow its owner everywhere.**"
— Chinese Proverb

Chapter 8
Linking ADDIE to Competency Frameworks

Competency frameworks, such as the ACGME Core Competencies, AACN Essentials, and LCME Standards, define the knowledge, skills, and attitudes required for healthcare professionals. These frameworks provide quality education and practice benchmarks, ensuring that training programs align with professional and institutional goals. When applied systematically, the ADDIE model can seamlessly integrate with these frameworks to create meaningful, competency-based healthcare simulations.

This chapter explores how each phase of the ADDIE model can incorporate competency frameworks, providing practical examples and strategies to align instructional design with professional standards.

1. Analysis Phase: Identifying Competency Gaps

The Analysis phase focuses on identifying learning needs and performance gaps. Competency frameworks serve as a reference point, helping educators and facilitators prioritize areas of improvement.

How to Integrate Competencies:

- **Review Competency Standards:** Identify relevant frameworks, such as ACGME milestones for medical residents or AACN Essentials for nursing students.
- **Conduct Data-Driven Needs Assessments:** Use clinical data, performance reviews, and learner feedback to pinpoint gaps relative to competencies.
- **Prioritize Training Needs:** Focus on high-impact competencies, such as patient safety, effective communication, or interprofessional collaboration.

Example:
In a hospital where patient handoffs frequently lead to errors, the Analysis phase identifies gaps in structured communication. Using the ACGME competency for **Interpersonal and Communication Skills**, the program prioritizes training on SBAR (Situation, Background, Assessment, Recommendation) handoff techniques.

2. Design Phase: Structuring Competency-Based Objectives

In the Design phase, learning objectives are developed to address the competencies identified during the Analysis phase. These objectives guide the creation of scenarios, activities, and assessments.

How to Integrate Competencies:

- **Map Objectives to Competencies:** Ensure each objective aligns with specific standards or milestones outlined in frameworks.
- **Incorporate Measurable Outcomes:** Use SMART (Specific, Measurable, Achievable, Relevant, Time-bound) objectives to define learner expectations clearly.
- **Plan Assessments:** Develop rubrics or checklists that directly measure competency achievement.

Example:
For a nursing simulation focusing on patient-centered care (AACN Essential VIII), the Design phase develops objectives like:

"Demonstrate culturally competent communication during a patient interview."

"Incorporate patient preferences into a care plan."

3. Development Phase: Building Competency-Based Resources

The Development phase involves creating materials, scenarios, and tools to achieve the objectives defined in the Design phase. Competency frameworks ensure that the content is accurate, relevant, and aligned with professional standards.

How to Integrate Competencies:

- **Collaborate with SMEs:** Subject matter experts validate clinical content and ensure alignment with evidence-based practices.
- **Focus on Realism:** Develop scenarios that reflect real-world challenges tied to competencies.
- **Pilot Test for Competency Alignment:** Ensure that materials effectively address the targeted skills and knowledge.

Example:
For a simulation targeting the ACGME competency of **Systems-Based Practice**, developers create a scenario in which learners navigate resource constraints during a mass casualty event. The materials emphasize teamwork, decision-making, and understanding healthcare systems.

4. Implementation Phase: Delivering Competency-Based Training

In the Implementation phase, simulations are conducted, and learners engage in activities designed to build and assess competencies. Facilitators play a key role in guiding learners and ensuring the training environment aligns with the intended outcomes.

How to Integrate Competencies:

- **Prepare Facilitators:** Train facilitators to emphasize competencies during simulations and debriefings.
- **Set Clear Expectations:** Provide learners with pre-simulation briefings that connect activities to specific competencies.
- **Ensure Real-Time Feedback:** Use structured tools to provide immediate feedback on competency-based performance.

Example:
During a simulation on managing acute myocardial infarction, facilitators highlight the ACGME competency for **Patient Care** by guiding learners to prioritize interventions like rapid ECG interpretation and timely medication administration.

5. Evaluation Phase: Measuring Competency Achievement

The Evaluation phase assesses whether learners have achieved the desired competencies and identifies areas for future improvement. This phase also measures the effectiveness of the simulation program in meeting institutional and professional standards.

How to Integrate Competencies:

- **Use Competency-Based Tools:** Apply rubrics, checklists, and performance metrics tied directly to competencies.
- **Gather Multi-Source Feedback:** Include evaluations from facilitators, peers, and learners to ensure a holistic assessment.
- **Analyze Outcomes:** Use data to determine whether learners meet competency benchmarks and adjust future training accordingly.

Example:
A sepsis management simulation evaluates learners on the AACN competency for **Evidence-Based Practice** by assessing their adherence to sepsis protocols, such as administering antibiotics within one hour of symptom recognition.

DESIGN, DEVELOP, DELIVER: USING ADDIE TO BUILD EFFECTIVE HEALTHCARE SIMULATIONS

Phase	How to Integrate Competencies
Analyze	• Identify relevant frameworks (e.g., ACGME, AACN, LCME) to guide the needs assessment. Use performance reviews and learner feedback to pinpoint gaps.
Design	• Map learning objectives to specific competencies. Develop measurable objectives and plan assessments aligned with professional standards.
Develop	• Collaborate with SMEs to create realistic, competency-driven scenarios. Ensure materials are evidence-based and reflect real-world challenges.
Implement	• Prepare facilitators to emphasize competencies during simulations. Provide real-time feedback and ensure activities align with the objectives.
Evaluate	• Use competency-based evaluation tools like rubrics and checklists. Gather feedback to determine whether competency benchmarks are achieved.

Key Takeaways

1. Competency Frameworks Provide Direction
    - Standards like ACGME milestones and AACN Essentials ensure that simulations target relevant, high-impact skills and knowledge.
2. Integration Enhances Alignment
    - By linking each phase of ADDIE to competencies, simulation programs align with accreditation requirements, institutional goals, and learner needs.
3. Realism Drives Relevance
    - Scenarios and activities grounded in competency frameworks reflect real-world challenges, enhancing learner engagement and preparedness.
4. Assessment Ensures Accountability
    - Competency-based tools and evaluation methods provide measurable evidence of learner achievement and program effectiveness.

Reflection

Competency frameworks are more than checklists—they are the foundation for creating meaningful, impactful training experiences. By embedding these standards into every phase of the ADDIE model, healthcare simulation programs can achieve alignment with professional expectations while delivering practical, engaging education.

As you reflect on your own simulation programs, consider the following:

- Are your learning objectives explicitly linked to competencies?
- Do your scenarios and materials reflect real-world challenges that align with professional standards?
- Are your assessments designed to measure competency achievement effectively?

By addressing these questions and adopting a competency-based approach, you ensure that your simulations meet educational goals and prepare learners to excel in their professional roles.

References

Accreditation Council for Graduate Medical Education (ACGME). (2022). *ACGME Common Program Requirements.* Retrieved from https://www.acgme.org

American Association of Colleges of Nursing (AACN). (2021). *The Essentials: Core competencies for professional nursing education.* Retrieved from https://www.aacnnursing.org

Branch, R. M. (2009). *Instructional design: The ADDIE approach.* Springer Science & Business Media.

Gagné, R. M., Wager, W. W., Golas, K. C., & Keller, J. M. (2005). *Principles of instructional design* (5th ed.). Wadsworth/Thomson Learning.

Liaison Committee on Medical Education (LCME). (2022). *Accreditation standards.* Retrieved from https://lcme.org

Morrison, G. R., Ross, S. M., Kalman, H. K., & Kemp, J. E. (2013). *Designing effective instruction* (7th ed.). Wiley.

Chapter 9
Iterative Refinement in the ADDIE Model

The ADDIE model is a cornerstone of instructional design, valued for its systematic and structured approach. However, in dynamic and fast-paced environments like healthcare simulation, its effectiveness lies in its adaptability rather than its linearity. Iterative refinement transforms the ADDIE model from a static framework into a responsive, evolving process. By embracing feedback loops between phases, simulation designers can enhance their training programs' relevance, realism, and impact.

This chapter delves into the concept of iterative refinement, highlighting how feedback and continuous improvement drive the success of healthcare simulations. Through detailed examples and actionable strategies, we explore how the ADDIE model evolves to meet healthcare education's complex and ever-changing needs.

Why Iterative Refinement Matters

Healthcare simulation is inherently dynamic. Learners' needs shift, clinical guidelines evolve, and organizational priorities change. A rigid, one-size-fits-all approach to instructional design cannot adequately address these complexities. Iterative refinement ensures that:

- **Simulations Stay Relevant**: Simulations evolve to reflect current clinical practices and challenges by continuously incorporating feedback.
- **Learning Outcomes Improve**: Refinements based on real-world performance data target gaps more effectively, resulting in better learner preparedness.
- **Flexibility Meets Reality**: The ability to revisit and revise earlier phases ensures the design process adapts to unforeseen challenges or opportunities.

Rather than viewing ADDIE as a step-by-step sequence, iterative refinement allows phases to interact fluidly. For example, insights from the Evaluation phase might inform changes in the Design phase, or challenges identified during Implementation may prompt updates to materials developed earlier. This flexibility is critical in high-stakes environments where training must be precise and responsive.

Feedback Loops in Action: Revisiting Phases

Evaluation to Design: Closing the Loop

The Evaluation phase offers a wealth of data on what works and what doesn't. Revisiting the Design phase based on these insights ensures that simulations are continuously improved.

Scenario:

A post-simulation evaluation for a trauma response scenario reveals that learners struggle with prioritizing tasks under pressure. Feedback indicates that the scenario lacks clarity in defining roles and responsibilities.

Refinement:

In the Design phase, learning objectives are updated to emphasize role clarity. The scenario script has been revised to include explicit task assignments and prompts that encourage learners to delegate effectively.

Implementation to Development: Real-Time Adjustments

During the Implementation phase, facilitators often identify practical issues that were not apparent during earlier stages. These insights inform refinements in the Development phase.

Scenario:
In a neonatal resuscitation simulation, facilitators notice that learners are confused by the equipment setup, leading to delays in initiating treatment.

Refinement:
Pre-simulation orientation materials are created in the Development phase to familiarize learners with the equipment. Additionally, the facilitator guide is updated to include troubleshooting tips.

Development to Design: Testing and Adjusting

Pilot testing during the Development phase often uncovers gaps in the initial design. Iterative refinement ensures these issues are addressed before full implementation.

Scenario:
During pilot testing for an ACLS (Advanced Cardiac Life Support) simulation, learners report feeling overwhelmed by the rapid pace of events.

Refinement:
The Design phase is revisited to stagger critical decision points, allowing learners more time to process information and respond. A practice round is added to build confidence before the main scenario.

Analysis to Evaluation: Informing Future Needs

Evaluation findings don't just improve current simulations—they also inform future needs assessments during the Analysis phase.

Scenario:
Evaluation data from a sepsis simulation reveals consistent gaps in recognizing early signs of patient deterioration. Facilitators and educators highlight this as a recurring issue.

Refinement:
During the next analysis phase, early recognition of clinical deterioration will be prioritized as a key training need. This leads to new simulations specifically targeting these skills.

Strategies for Effective Iterative Refinement

1. **Create Structured Feedback Mechanisms**
   - Collect feedback from facilitators, learners, and SMEs during and after each phase.
   - Use surveys, focus groups, and debriefing sessions to gather actionable insights.

2. **Prioritize Collaboration**
   - Engage stakeholders in regular review sessions to discuss findings and plan refinements.
   - Foster a culture where feedback is welcomed and acted upon.

3. **Leverage Technology**
   - Use learning management systems (LMS) to track learner performance trends and identify areas for improvement.
   - Incorporate simulation analytics to measure specific behaviors, such as reaction times or decision accuracy.

4. **Test Changes Incrementally**

- Pilot-test updates with small groups before implementing them at scale.
- Evaluate the effectiveness of changes and refine further based on feedback.

5. **Document Revisions**
   - Maintain detailed records of changes, including the rationale and outcomes.
   - Use documentation to inform future simulations and prevent recurring issues.

Case Studies: Iterative Refinement in Practice

Case Study 1: Sepsis Management Simulation
Initial Issue:
Post-simulation evaluations reveal that learners fail to recognize subtle signs of sepsis in a timely manner.
Refinement:
The scenario is redesigned to include clearer cues, such as changes in patient vitals and audible prompts. Facilitators are trained to provide hints during critical moments. Subsequent evaluations show improved learner performance.

Case Study 2: Team Communication Training
Initial Issue:
Facilitators report that learners struggle with effective communication during a trauma team simulation, leading to confusion and delays.
Refinement:
A new pre-simulation exercise on closed-loop communication is added, and role assignments are made more explicit in the scenario. Pilot testing confirms enhanced teamwork and coordination.

Case Study 3: Medication Safety Scenario
Initial Issue:
Learners miss critical steps in the "five rights" of medication administration due to distractions in the simulation environment.
Refinement:
A pre-simulation briefing is introduced to focus on managing

interruptions. The scenario is adjusted to include periodic reminders, and rubrics are updated to assess learners' responses to distractions.

Benefits of Iterative Refinement

Enhanced Relevance
Continuous updates ensure that simulations reflect current clinical guidelines and organizational priorities.

Improved Learner Outcomes
Targeted refinements address specific gaps, resulting in more effective training and better preparation for real-world challenges.

Increased Stakeholder Engagement
Involving stakeholders in feedback loops fosters a sense of ownership and ensures diverse perspectives are considered.

Sustainability
Iterative refinement helps programs adapt to changing needs, ensuring long-term value and impact.

Iterative refinement is not just an enhancement to the ADDIE model—it is essential for its success in dynamic environments like healthcare simulation. By embracing feedback loops, instructional designers can create simulations that evolve with learner needs, clinical practices, and organizational goals. The iterative nature of ADDIE transforms it into a powerful, adaptive tool, ensuring that every simulation is impactful and continuously improving. Through structured feedback, collaboration, and real-world testing, iterative refinement is key to delivering meaningful, lasting learning experiences.

Takeaways

1. Iterative Refinement Enhances ADDIE's Adaptability
   - The ADDIE model is most effective when treated as a dynamic, cyclic process. Iterative refinement allows for continuous improvements by revisiting earlier phases based on feedback and real-world insights.

2. Feedback Loops Are Essential for Improvement
   - Evaluation informs Design, Implementation identifies Development gaps, and insights from all phases guide Analysis for future iterations. Feedback loops ensure every phase contributes to better outcomes.
3. Collaboration Drives Refinement
   - Stakeholders, including educators, facilitators, SMEs, and learners, play pivotal roles in providing actionable feedback. Their diverse perspectives ensure the refinement process addresses all critical aspects.
4. Real-World Testing is Critical
   - Pilot testing and phased implementation reveal practical challenges, allowing for targeted refinements before scaling. Incremental changes driven by real-world data lead to more effective simulations.
5. Documentation Supports Continuous Improvement
   - Detailed records of changes and their outcomes create a valuable resource for future projects, preventing repeated errors and ensuring lessons learned are applied.
6. Healthcare-Specific Benefits
   - In healthcare simulation, iterative refinement ensures that scenarios remain clinically accurate, relevant, and aligned with professional standards, ultimately improving patient care outcomes.

Reflection

Iterative refinement is the engine that transforms the ADDIE model from a static framework into a dynamic tool for continuous improvement. Healthcare simulation, with its high stakes and evolving challenges, demands this adaptability. Reflecting on the iterative nature of ADDIE reveals how powerful feedback loops can bridge the gap between theoretical design and practical application.

As you consider iterative refinement in your projects, ask yourself:
- Are you collecting actionable feedback at every phase, and from all stakeholders?

- Do your refinement processes allow for quick adjustments without compromising quality?
- How well do your simulations evolve to reflect changes in clinical guidelines, learner needs, and organizational priorities?

By embedding iterative refinement into the ADDIE process, you ensure that every simulation becomes a steppingstone to better training, stronger outcomes, and improved patient care. It's not just about delivering effective simulations—it's about creating a culture of excellence that continuously adapts and grows.

Resources

Branch, R. M. (2009). *Instructional design: The ADDIE approach*. Springer Science & Business Media.

Dick, W., Carey, L., & Carey, J. O. (2015). *The systematic design of instruction* (8th ed.). Pearson.

Gagné, R. M., Wager, W. W., Golas, K. C., & Keller, J. M. (2005). *Principles of instructional design* (5th ed.). Wadsworth/Thomson Learning.

Hodell, C. (2016). *ISD: From the ground up: A concise introduction to instructional design* (4th ed.). American Society for Training and Development.

Kirkpatrick, D. L., & Kirkpatrick, J. D. (2006). *Evaluating training programs: The four levels*. Berrett-Koehler Publishers.

Morrison, G. R., Ross, S. M., Kalman, H. K., & Kemp, J. E. (2013). *Designing effective instruction* (7th ed.). Wiley.

Rosen, M. A., Hunt, E. A., Pronovost, P. J., Federowicz, M. A., & Weaver, S. J. (2012). In situ simulation in continuing education for the healthcare professions: A systematic review. *Journal of Continuing Education in the Health Professions, 32*(4), 243–254. https://doi.org/10.1002/chp.21152

Svinicki, M. D., & McKeachie, W. J. (2014). *McKeachie's teaching tips: Strategies, research, and theory for college and university teachers* (14th ed.). Wadsworth Cengage Learning.

Zigmont, J. J., Kappus, L. J., & Sudikoff, S. N. (2011). The 3D model of debriefing: Defusing, discovering, and deepening. *Seminars in Perinatology, 35*(2), 52–58. https://doi.org/10.1053/j.semperi.2011.01.003

Chapter 10
Scaling Simulations Across Learner Levels

Healthcare learners come from diverse backgrounds with varying experience, knowledge, and skills. A one-size-fits-all approach to simulation training may fall short of meeting these unique needs. Scaling simulations across learner levels—novice, intermediate, and advanced—ensures that training is appropriately challenging, impactful, and aligned with individual competencies.

This chapter explores the principles and strategies for tailoring healthcare simulations to different learner levels, providing actionable insights and examples to guide instructional design.

The Importance of Scaling Simulations

Scaling simulations offers several benefits:
- **Individualized Learning**: Tailoring scenarios ensures that learners focus on skills relevant to their current proficiency level.
- **Progressive Skill Development**: Gradually increasing complexity allows learners to build foundational knowledge before tackling advanced challenges.

- **Maximized Engagement**: Simulations that align with learners' abilities prevent boredom for advanced participants and overwhelm for novices.
- **Competency Alignment**: Scaled simulations better align with frameworks like the ACGME Core Competencies or AACN Essentials.

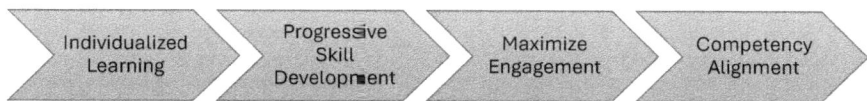

Importance of Scaling Simulations

Framework for Scaling Simulations Across Learner Levels

1. Analyze Phase: Identifying Learner Needs

The Analysis phase determines the current proficiency level of learners and their specific training needs.
- **Novice Learners**: Focus on foundational gaps, such as basic clinical knowledge and procedural skills.
- **Intermediate Learners**: Identify areas where learners can integrate skills, such as applying knowledge in moderately complex situations.
- **Advanced Learners**: Target higher-order skills like leadership, decision-making, and managing unpredictable scenarios.

Example:
For a sepsis management program:
- Novices may lack basic knowledge of sepsis protocols.
- Intermediates need practice prioritizing interventions.
- Advanced learners may require scenarios involving interdisciplinary teamwork under time pressure.

2. Design Phase: Creating Scaled Objectives
In the Design phase, learning objectives are crafted to match the complexity of each learner level.
- **Novice Objectives**: Focus on skill acquisition and knowledge application.

  Example: "Recognize early signs of sepsis and initiate treatment within 10 minutes."

- **Intermediate Objectives**: Emphasize integration of skills and decision-making.

  Example: "Prioritize interventions based on a patient's condition during a sepsis crisis."

- **Advanced Objectives**: Address leadership, adaptability, and advanced clinical reasoning.

  Example: "Lead a multidisciplinary team in managing a patient with septic shock and resource constraints."

3. Development Phase: Building Scaled Resources
The Development phase involves creating scenarios, tools, and materials tailored to each learner level.

Novice Resources:
- Guided scripts and detailed facilitator guides.
- Low-fidelity tools (e.g., basic mannequins, role-playing).

Intermediate Resources:
- Moderate-fidelity simulations with decision points.
- Scenarios integrating teamwork and moderately complex cases.

Advanced Resources:
- High-fidelity simulations with branching pathways and unpredictable variables.
- Multidisciplinary and interprofessional scenarios.

Example:
For a trauma response simulation:
- Novices practice initial stabilization techniques using basic mannequins.
- Intermediates manage a deteriorating patient with time-sensitive interventions.
- Advanced learners handle complex trauma cases involving multiple injuries and resource limitations.

4. Implementation Phase: Tailored Facilitation
Facilitators are critical in ensuring that simulations match the learner's level and provide appropriate guidance.

Novice Learners:
- High facilitator involvement with step-by-step guidance.
- Frequent feedback during the simulation.

Intermediate Learners:
- Limited facilitator intervention, encouraging learner autonomy.
- Focus on building confidence in decision-making.

Advanced Learners:
- Minimal facilitator involvement, emphasizing independent leadership.
- Debriefing focused on advanced reflection and critical analysis.

5. Evaluation Phase: Measuring Scaled Outcomes
The Evaluation phase ensures that assessments align with learner levels, providing meaningful feedback.

Novice Learners:
- Use checklists focusing on task completion and adherence to protocols.
- Provide detailed feedback to reinforce foundational skills.

Intermediate Learners:
- Use rubrics to assess the integration of technical and non-technical skills.
- Encourage peer and self-assessment for reflective learning.

Advanced Learners:
- Employ comprehensive evaluations assessing leadership, adaptability, and team dynamics.
- Use summative assessments aligned with professional competencies.

Example:
For a communication-focused simulation:
- Novices are assessed on clarity and accuracy in delivering SBAR reports.
- Intermediates are evaluated on communication and prioritization under moderate stress.
- Advanced learners are assessed on managing team communication during a high-pressure multidisciplinary case.

Template for Scaling Simulations

Phase	Novice Learners	Intermediate Learners	Advanced Learners
Analyze	- Focus on foundational knowledge gaps (e.g., basic skills, terminology). - Identify confidence barriers and misconceptions. - Engage stakeholders to determine basic competency needs.	- Target specific skills and knowledge gaps, such as application of concepts. - Assess moderate proficiency in technical and non-technical areas. - Identify common challenges in real-world applications.	- Address advanced competencies, such as leadership, decision-making, and handling complex scenarios. - Use performance data to pinpoint gaps in mastery and refinement needs. - Explore interprofessional collaboration opportunities.
Design	- Create SMART objectives focusing on fundamental skills and knowledge. - Use structured, step-by-step scenarios with clear	- Develop objectives targeting integration of technical and non-technical skills. - Use moderately complex scenarios with decision	- Craft objectives addressing advanced problem-solving and critical thinking. - Design high-pressure, multidisciplinary

Phase	Novice Learners	Intermediate Learners	Advanced Learners
	guidance. - Incorporate frequent checkpoints for feedback.	points. - Include teamwork and communication objectives.	scenarios requiring leadership and adaptability. - Incorporate unpredictable variables to enhance realism.
Develop	- Build resources such as guided scripts, detailed facilitator guides, and step-by-step task checklists. - Use low-to-moderate fidelity simulations (e.g., basic mannequins, role-playing). - Emphasize structured debriefing templates.	- Create intermediate scenarios integrating realistic decision-making and moderate fidelity tools (e.g., partial task trainers, electronic monitors). - Develop facilitator prompts for supporting semi-independent learners.	- Develop high-fidelity simulations with advanced tools (e.g., VR/AR environments, fully programmed mannequins). - Include branching scenarios to mimic real-world complexities. - Use advanced debriefing strategies like root cause analysis.
Implement	- Provide significant facilitator guidance during scenarios. - Focus on skill acquisition and confidence-building. - Use shorter, highly focused simulation sessions.	- Allow learners to perform with minimal guidance, focusing on integrating skills. - Use moderate-length simulations that challenge decision-making. - Facilitate group-based learning experiences.	- Let learners take full control of scenarios, focusing on leadership and teamwork. - Use extended simulations that simulate full shifts or multidisciplinary case management. - Incorporate interprofessional team training.
Evaluate	- Use formative assessments like observation checklists and facilitator feedback. - Focus on individual progress in achieving basic	- Employ rubrics assessing both technical and non-technical skills. - Use peer and self-assessment to encourage reflection.	- Use comprehensive evaluations measuring leadership, decision-making, and outcomes. - Focus on

Phase	Novice Learners	Intermediate Learners	Advanced Learners
	competencies. - Provide detailed, supportive feedback post-simulation.	- Identify trends to guide ongoing learning.	summative assessments aligned with professional competencies. - Collect longitudinal data to track advanced skill development.

Case Study: Scaling a Cardiac Arrest Simulation

Scenario Overview:

A cardiac arrest simulation is tailored for novice, intermediate, and advanced learners.

Novice Simulation:

- Focus: Basic CPR technique and AED use.
- Scenario: Single patient collapse in a controlled setting.

Intermediate Simulation:

- Focus: ACLS protocol integration and team communication.
- Scenario: Patient decompensating with multiple team members involved.

Advanced Simulation:

- Focus: Team leadership, decision-making, and handling resource constraints.
- Scenario: Cardiac arrest during a mass casualty event.

Benefits of Scaling Simulations

- **Tailored Learning Experiences**
  Simulations match the learner's skill level, ensuring engagement and appropriate challenges.

- **Improved Competency Development**

Learners progress from foundational skills to advanced proficiencies in a structured manner.

- **Enhanced Realism and Relevance**
  Scenarios evolve to reflect real-world challenges as learners advance.

- **Efficient Resource Utilization**
  Tools and materials are adapted to maximize their impact across learner levels.

Key Takeaways

1. Scalability Meets Diverse Needs
   - Scaling simulations ensures training is relevant and impactful for learners at all proficiency levels.
2. Structured Progression Enhances Learning
   - Gradually increasing complexity builds confidence and mastery over time.
3. Alignment with Competencies
   - Scaled simulations align with frameworks like ACGME and AACN, ensuring professional standards are met.
4. Facilitators Drive Tailored Experiences
   - Adjusting facilitation styles to learner levels enhances engagement and autonomy.

Reflection

Scaling simulations require thoughtful planning and execution but offers immense value in healthcare education. Reflecting on your current simulations, consider:

- Are your simulations appropriately challenging for all learners?
- Do you provide progressive learning experiences that align with professional competencies?
- Are your evaluations tailored to measure success at different proficiency levels?

By addressing these questions and implementing scalable strategies, you can create simulations that foster growth, confidence, and excellence at every stage of a learner's journey.

References

American Association of Colleges of Nursing (AACN). (2021). *The Essentials: Core competencies for professional nursing education.* Retrieved from https://www.aacnnursing.org

Branch, R. M. (2009). *Instructional design: The ADDIE approach.* Springer Science & Business Media.

Gagné, R. M., Wager, W. W., Golas, K. C., & Keller, J. M. (2005). *Principles of instructional design* (5th ed.). Wadsworth/Thomson Learning.

Morrison, G. R., Ross, S. M., Kalman, H. K., & Kemp, J. E. (2013). *Designing effective instruction* (7th ed.). Wiley.

Accreditation Council for Graduate Medical Education (ACGME). (2022). *ACGME Common Program Requirements.* Retrieved from https://www.acgme.org

"Learning is not attained by chance, it must be sought for with ardor and attended to with diligence."
— Abigail Adams

Chapter 11
Interdisciplinary Applications of the ADDIE Model

Modern healthcare's complexity demands clinical expertise and the ability to work seamlessly across disciplines. Effective collaboration is critical to ensuring patient safety and improving outcomes, from physicians to nurses to pharmacists and administrators. However, many training programs focus primarily on individual competencies, overlooking the need for interdisciplinary skills like teamwork, communication, leadership, and systems thinking.

This chapter expands on how the ADDIE model can be used to design and implement interdisciplinary simulations, emphasizing their role in preparing healthcare professionals for the collaborative challenges of real-world practice. By leveraging the structured approach of ADDIE, educators can create dynamic, competency-driven simulations that foster teamwork and shared accountability.

The Need for Interdisciplinary Simulations

Healthcare delivery is inherently interprofessional, involving diverse teams with distinct but overlapping roles. However, ineffective communication, unclear expectations, and power imbalances within teams often lead to errors and inefficiencies. Interdisciplinary simulations address these issues by:

- **Promoting Mutual Understanding:** Helping team members appreciate the unique contributions of each role.
- **Enhancing Collaboration:** Developing skills to navigate complex team dynamics and achieve shared goals.
- **Building Leadership and Systems Thinking:** Preparing participants to take initiative and make decisions in high-pressure, multi-stakeholder situations.

Interdisciplinary simulations create a safe environment for learners to practice these skills, bridging the gap between individual expertise and team-based care.

Applying ADDIE to Interdisciplinary Simulations

The ADDIE model provides a structured yet flexible framework for designing interdisciplinary simulations. Each phase of ADDIE offers opportunities to align training with the unique demands of team-based healthcare.

1. Analyze Phase: Identifying Gaps in Team Dynamics

The Analyze phase is crucial for understanding the challenges that interdisciplinary teams face. Unlike individual-focused simulations, this phase emphasizes team-based performance, interprofessional collaboration, and systems-based challenges.

Key Activities:
- Conduct surveys and focus groups with interdisciplinary teams to identify common pain points.
- Observe real-world interactions to assess communication patterns and role clarity.
- Review incident reports or patient safety metrics data to pinpoint systemic issues.

Example:
A hospital experiencing delays in medication reconciliation during patient discharges conducts focus groups with nursing, pharmacy, and medical teams. The analysis reveals inconsistent communication and

unclear role expectations, setting the stage for a simulation focused on collaborative workflows.

2. Design Phase: Crafting Team-Centric Objectives

The Design phase involves translating the insights from the analysis phase into structured, measurable objectives emphasizing teamwork and collaboration.

Key Considerations:
- Define objectives that reflect the competencies required for effective team performance, such as ACGME's **Interpersonal and Communication Skills** or AACN's **Interprofessional Collaboration.**
- Develop scenarios that mimic real-world challenges, requiring input and coordination from multiple roles.
- Plan assessments that evaluate team dynamics shared decision-making, and role clarity.

Example Objectives for a Leadership Simulation:
- "Facilitate a team discussion to prioritize patient needs during a resource shortage."
- "Resolve interprofessional conflicts to maintain focus on patient safety."

3. Development Phase: Building Scenarios for Collaboration

The Development phase brings the design to life by creating scenarios, materials, and tools tailored to interdisciplinary contexts. This phase emphasizes realism and role-specific challenges.

Key Activities:
- Develop scenarios that require input from multiple disciplines, such as responding to a mass casualty incident or managing a chronic disease in a community setting.
- Create role-specific briefs that outline each participant's responsibilities and expertise.
- Pilot test scenarios to ensure they reflect real-world complexity and promote meaningful collaboration.

- *Example:*
  For a simulation addressing system failures during a hospital power outage, the development process includes:
  - Designing scenarios where nurses ensure patient safety, pharmacists safeguard medication, and administrators coordinate logistics.
  - Testing these scenarios with small pilot groups to identify gaps and refine the materials.

4. Implementation Phase: Guiding Team Learning

Implementation is where the simulation is delivered to interdisciplinary teams. Effective facilitation ensures that participants engage fully and learn from the experience.

Facilitator Role:
- Encourage equal participation from all team members, addressing power imbalances or conflicts as they arise.
- Guide teams through complex scenarios while allowing them to own decisions.
- Use prompts to highlight critical moments and encourage reflective thinking.

Learner Preparation:
- Provide a pre-simulation briefing that emphasizes the importance of collaboration and outlines the scenario's goals.
- Clarify the value of each team member's role in achieving shared outcomes.

Example:
During a simulation on managing patient handoffs, facilitators ensure that physicians, nurses, and pharmacists contribute their expertise. The debriefing focuses on the impact of effective communication and role clarity on patient safety.

5. Evaluation Phase: Measuring Interprofessional Success

The Evaluation phase assesses how well the simulation achieved its goals and identifies opportunities for improvement. It emphasizes team-based metrics rather than individual performance alone.

Key Activities:
- Use rubrics that evaluate team communication, conflict resolution, and shared decision-making.
- Gather feedback from participants and facilitators to identify strengths and areas for refinement.
- Analyze long-term impacts, such as improved team dynamics or better patient outcomes.

Example:
Evaluations after a leadership simulation show significant improvements in participants' ability to mediate conflicts and prioritize patient safety during emergencies. Follow-up surveys confirm sustained confidence in addressing interprofessional challenges.

Phase	Key Activities
Analyze	- Conduct surveys and focus groups with interdisciplinary teams to identify common pain points. - Observe real-world interactions to assess communication patterns and role clarity. - Review data from incident reports or patient safety metrics to pinpoint systemic issues.
Design	- Define objectives reflecting competencies like ACGME's Interpersonal and Communication Skills or AACN's Interprofessional Collaboration. - Develop scenarios requiring coordination across multiple roles. - Plan assessments for team dynamics, shared decision-making, and role clarity.
Develop	- Develop scenarios requiring input from multiple disciplines, such as mass casualty response or chronic disease management. - Create role-specific briefs outlining responsibilities and expertise. - Pilot test scenarios for realism and collaboration.
Implement	- Encourage equal participation and address power imbalances. - Guide teams through scenarios while allowing independent decision-making. - Use prompts to highlight critical moments and encourage reflection.
Evaluate	- Use rubrics to evaluate communication, conflict resolution, and shared decision-making. - Collect feedback from participants and facilitators.

	- Analyze long-term impacts like improved team dynamics and patient outcomes.

Case Study: Interprofessional Collaboration for Patient Safety

Scenario Overview:
A simulation is designed to improve collaboration between nursing, medical, and pharmacy teams during medication reconciliation.

Analyze Phase: Focus groups reveal that inconsistent communication leads to delays and errors.

Design Phase: Objectives include "demonstrate effective communication during medication handoffs" and "clarify team roles and responsibilities."

Development Phase: A realistic scenario is created where nurses, physicians, and pharmacists must work together to reconcile a complex medication list.

Implementation Phase: Teams engage in the simulation, guided by facilitators who address power imbalances and emphasize shared accountability.

Evaluation Phase: Rubrics measure team communication and conflict resolution. Post-simulation feedback highlights improved collaboration and understanding of roles.

Key Takeaways

1. Teamwork and Collaboration Are Essential
   - Interdisciplinary simulations prepare healthcare professionals to navigate complex team dynamics and shared decision-making.
2. Competency Frameworks Provide Structure
   - Aligning simulations with standards like ACGME's **Systems-Based Practice** or AACN's **Interprofessional Collaboration** ensures relevance and rigor.
3. Facilitators Are Critical

- Skilled facilitation ensures that all voices are heard and that simulations achieve their full potential.
4. Feedback Drives Improvement
    - Evaluations provide actionable insights for refining scenarios and addressing team-based challenges.

Reflection

Healthcare delivery depends on the strength of its teams. Interdisciplinary simulations bridge the gap between individual competencies and collaborative practice, preparing learners for the complexities of real-world care. As you consider your simulation programs, reflect on the following:

- Are your scenarios designed to promote interprofessional collaboration?
- Do your objectives emphasize team-based outcomes?
- Are you equipping facilitators to manage diverse teams effectively?

By addressing these questions and applying the ADDIE model to interdisciplinary contexts, you can create simulations that enhance teamwork, leadership, and systems thinking across healthcare disciplines.

References

American Association of Colleges of Nursing (AACN). (2021). *The Essentials: Core competencies for professional nursing education.* Retrieved from https://www.aacnnursing.org

Branch, R. M. (2009). *Instructional design: The ADDIE approach.* Springer Science & Business Media.

Gagné, R. M., Wager, W. W., Golas, K. C., & Keller, J. M. (2005). *Principles of instructional design* (5th ed.). Wadsworth/Thomson Learning.

Morrison, G. R., Ross, S. M., Kalman, H. K., & Kemp, J. E. (2013). *Designing effective instruction* (7th ed.). Wiley.

Accreditation Council for Graduate Medical Education (ACGME). (2022). *ACGME Common Program Requirements.* Retrieved from https://www.acgme.org

"Wisdom is not a product of schooling but of the lifelong attempt to acquire it."
— Albert Einstein

DESIGN, DEVELOP, DELIVER: USING ADDIE TO BUILD EFFECTIVE
HEALTHCARE SIMULATIONS

Chapter 12
Case Studies

The beauty of the ADDIE model lies in its universality and adaptability. Across healthcare settings—be it a bustling trauma center, a small community clinic, or an academic classroom—the model provides a structured yet flexible framework for designing impactful simulation programs. By examining real-world applications of ADDIE, we can uncover how its principles are put into practice, adapt it to specific contexts, and learn from both successes and challenges.

This chapter highlights case studies that illustrate the power of ADDIE in healthcare simulation. Each story reflects not only how the model transforms learning but also how it navigates unique challenges and fosters growth. Through these examples, we'll explore successes, lessons learned, and strategies for adapting ADDIE to diverse settings.

Success Stories

Case Study 1: Enhancing Team Communication in Emergency Trauma Care

Setting: A Level 1 trauma center managing high-acuity patients in a fast-paced environment

Objective: Improve interprofessional communication and decision-making during trauma resuscitations.

The Challenge:
Frequent breakdowns in team communication led to delays in patient care during trauma cases. Staff feedback revealed role confusion and inconsistent use of closed-loop communication strategies.

ADDIE in Action:
- **Analysis:** Data from incident reports, focus groups, and team surveys highlighted communication issues as the primary barrier to effective trauma care. The analysis revealed that staff needed more practice in structured communication and role clarity during emergencies.
- **Design:** The curriculum focused on scenarios that required teams to handle critical events such as hypotension and multi-organ trauma. Learning objectives emphasized closed-loop communication, role assignment, and rapid information exchange.
- **Development:** High-fidelity mannequins, simulated trauma bays, and standardized patients were integrated into the scenarios. Facilitator guides outlined key triggers, like sudden patient deterioration, to challenge learners and assess communication under stress.
- **Implementation:** Interdisciplinary teams, including physicians, nurses, and respiratory therapists, participated in simulations. Sessions were followed by structured debriefings where facilitators used the "Defuse, Discover, Deepen" model to explore communication dynamics.
- **Evaluation:** Post-simulation surveys revealed a 35% improvement in participant confidence regarding communication skills. Real-world metrics showed a 20% reduction in time-to-intervention during actual trauma cases.

Key Takeaway:
The trauma center achieved measurable improvements in patient outcomes and team dynamics by identifying a specific problem and tailoring every phase of ADDIE to address it.

Case Study 2: Reducing Medication Errors in a Community Hospital

Setting: A community hospital with limited training resources

Objective: Reduce medication administration errors by empowering nurses with safer practices.

The Challenge:
Medication errors were identified as a persistent issue, with staff citing distractions and unclear protocols as contributing factors. Limited training resources required creative solutions.

ADDIE in Action:
- **Analysis:** Incident reports revealed recurring errors in dosage and timing. Focus groups with nursing staff identified a need for strategies to handle interruptions and verify medication accuracy.
- **Design:** Scenarios simulated real-world challenges, such as administering medications while managing a busy ward. Objectives emphasized safety checks, effective communication, and prioritization during interruptions.
- **Development:** Low-fidelity mannequins and simple props, such as mock medication labels and patient charts, were used. Facilitator guides included cues to introduce distractions, like call bells or patient questions.
- **Implementation:** Simulations were integrated into regular training sessions. Participants practiced using checklists and the "five rights" of medication administration in high-distraction environments.
- **Evaluation:** Post-training assessments showed a 25% decrease in medication errors over six months. Staff surveys indicated increased confidence in managing interruptions and adhering to safety protocols.

Key Takeaway:
Even with resource constraints, the ADDIE model can deliver impactful results by focusing on practical, targeted solutions.

Case Study 3: Building Cultural Competence in Community Health Workers

Setting: A community health center serving a multilingual, multicultural population

Objective: Enhance cultural competence and communication skills among health workers.

The Challenge:
Health workers struggled to address cultural barriers, leading to misunderstandings and reduced patient trust. Patients reported feeling unheard or misunderstood, impacting their adherence to care plans.

ADDIE in Action:
- **Analysis:** Surveys and interviews with patients and staff highlighted the need for improved communication strategies and cultural awareness. Common challenges included language barriers and differing healthcare beliefs.
- **Design:** Role-play scenarios were created to focus on empathy, active listening, and navigating cultural sensitivities. Objectives emphasized building rapport and tailoring care to individual patient needs.
- **Development:** Scenarios were based on real-life cases, such as addressing vaccine hesitancy or explaining chronic disease management in culturally appropriate ways. Community members acted as standardized patients to ensure authenticity.
- **Implementation:** Small group sessions allowed participants to practice their skills in a safe environment. Facilitators provided real-time feedback and led debriefings to explore cultural nuances and communication strategies.
- **Evaluation:** Patient satisfaction scores increased by 40%, and appointment no-show rates decreased. Staff reported feeling more confident addressing cultural challenges and building stronger patient relationships.

Key Takeaway:

The ADDIE model's flexibility allowed the health center to create a curriculum tailored to its unique patient population, fostering greater trust and improved outcomes.

Lessons Learned

From these success stories, we can draw important lessons about what makes the ADDIE model effective and how to navigate challenges during implementation:
1. **Start with Clear, Actionable Objectives:** A focused analysis phase ensures the curriculum addresses specific, measurable goals. For example, the trauma center targeted communication as a key area for improvement.
2. **Involve Stakeholders:** Engaging learners, facilitators, and even patients in the planning process ensures the curriculum meets real-world needs. The cultural competence program benefited from input by community members.
3. **Pilot Testing Matters:** Iterative testing during the Development Phase allows teams to identify and address gaps. In the medication safety program, pilot tests revealed that scenarios needed clearer instructions.
4. **Adapt to Resource Constraints:** Creativity can overcome budgetary limitations. The community hospital achieved significant results with low-cost props and role-play scenarios.
5. **Iterate and Improve:** Post-simulation feedback is invaluable for refining scenarios and addressing unforeseen issues, as demonstrated in all three case studies.

Adaptations for Specific Contexts

The ADDIE model is not a one-size-fits-all solution. Its strength lies in its ability to adapt to the unique needs of different healthcare settings.

Acute Care Settings
In high-stakes environments like emergency departments or ICUs:
- **Focus:** Rapid decision-making, teamwork, and critical thinking under pressure.

- **Adaptation:** Use high-fidelity mannequins and advanced monitoring systems to replicate real-life emergencies. Incorporate time-sensitive scenarios to simulate the urgency of acute care.

Community Health Settings
In community health, where relationships and communication are key:
- **Focus:** Building trust, addressing cultural differences, and promoting preventive care.
- **Adaptation:** Use role-play and case studies to address common challenges, such as explaining complex diagnoses to patients with limited health literacy.

Educational Programs
In academic settings, where learners are building foundational skills:
- **Focus:** Mastering technical skills, understanding protocols, and fostering clinical judgment.
- **Adaptation:** Create scaffolded simulations that build complexity over time, starting with basic skills and progressing to integrated scenarios.

Key Takeaways
1. The ADDIE model's structured approach enables programs to address specific challenges with tailored solutions.
2. Successful implementation depends on stakeholder engagement, realistic scenarios, and a commitment to continuous improvement.
3. Adaptations allow ADDIE to thrive in diverse healthcare settings, from acute care hospitals to community clinics.
4. Lessons learned from real-world examples highlight the importance of flexibility, creativity, and iterative refinement.

Reflection
Consider how the ADDIE model could address challenges in your own organization:
- What specific problems could be tackled using its structured approach?

- How can you engage stakeholders to create meaningful, relevant scenarios?
- What lessons from these case studies resonate most with your own practice?

By tailoring the ADDIE model to the unique needs of healthcare learners, we can build simulation programs that not only educate but also inspire lasting change and improved patient care.

References

Branch, R. M. (2009). *Instructional design: The ADDIE approach*. Springer Science & Business Media.

Fanning, R. M., & Gaba, D. M. (2007). The role of debriefing in simulation-based learning. *Simulation in Healthcare, 2*(2), 115–125. https://doi.org/10.1097/SIH.0b013e3180315539

Gaba, D. M. (2004). The future vision of simulation in healthcare. *Quality and Safety in Health Care, 13*(Suppl 1), i2–i10. https://doi.org/10.1136/qshc.2004.009878

Jeffries, P. R. (2012). Simulation in nursing education: From conceptualization to evaluation. *National League for Nursing*.

Kolb, D. A. (1984). *Experiential learning: Experience as the source of learning and development*. Prentice Hall.

Rosen, M. A., Salas, E., Silvestri, S., Wu, T. S., & Lazzara, E. H. (2008). Promoting teamwork: An event-based approach to simulation-based teamwork training for emergency medicine residents. *Academic Emergency Medicine, 15*(11), 1190–1198. https://doi.org/10.1111/j.1553-2712.2008.00243.x

Zigmont, J. J., Kappus, L. J., & Sudikoff, S. N. (2011). The 3D model of debriefing: Defusing, discovering, and deepening. *Seminars in Perinatology, 35*(2), 52–58. https://doi.org/10.1053/j.semperi.2011.01.003

"Every day is an opportunity to learn something new."
— Unknown

Chapter 13
Criticisms of the ADDIE Model for Healthcare Simulation and Adaptations for Flexibility

The ADDIE model—Analyze, Design, Develop, Implement, Evaluate—has long been a cornerstone of instructional design, praised for its systematic approach to creating effective training programs. However, its linear and structured nature can pose challenges when applied to the dynamic and often high-pressure field of healthcare simulation. The healthcare environment demands responsiveness to rapidly evolving needs, resource constraints, and diverse learner groups. These realities have led to criticisms of ADDIE and the need for adaptations to make it more applicable and efficient in healthcare simulation contexts.

In this chapter, we'll explore the primary criticisms of using the ADDIE model in healthcare simulation and offer practical ways to modify and optimize it to suit the unique demands of healthcare education better.

Criticisms of the ADDIE Model in Healthcare Simulation

1. Linear and Time-Consuming Process

One of the most frequent criticisms of ADDIE is its sequential, step-by-step approach. Each phase—Analyze, Design, Develop, Implement, and Evaluate—is traditionally completed before moving to the next, which can result in a lengthy timeline. This can be a significant drawback in healthcare simulation, where urgent training needs may arise.

Example: During a global health crisis like the COVID-19 pandemic, hospitals may need to train staff on new protocols for ventilator management quickly. Waiting to complete the Analyze and Design phases before starting Development and Implementation might delay critical training.

Impact: The linear process can feel inflexible and ill-suited to situations requiring rapid deployment of training programs.

2. Limited Flexibility

The structured nature of ADDIE can make it difficult to adapt mid-process. If new insights arise during Implementation, such as unexpected learner challenges, addressing them often requires revisiting earlier phases, which can disrupt the project's flow.

Example: In a trauma simulation, facilitators may notice that learners struggle with situational awareness, a skill not emphasized in the initial design. Modifying the simulation in real time can be difficult without a framework for adaptability.

3. Resource-Heavy Demands

The ADDIE model is resource-intensive, requiring significant time, personnel, and materials, particularly during the Analysis and Development phases. This can be a barrier for smaller healthcare facilities or programs operating on tight budgets.

Example: A rural hospital aiming to implement a simulation-based training program for obstetric emergencies may lack the staff or funds to conduct a thorough needs analysis or develop high-fidelity scenarios.

4. Overemphasis on Front-End Analysis
While the Analysis phase is crucial for identifying learning needs and setting objectives, critics argue that ADDIE's traditional approach places too much emphasis on this stage, potentially delaying action when immediate training is needed.

Example: A hospital may need immediate training for nurses in response to an increase in medication errors. Spending weeks gathering data and conducting interviews during the Analysis phase could delay timely intervention.

5. Perceived Rigidity in Real-world Application
In the fast-paced world of healthcare, where unexpected challenges are common, ADDIE's perceived rigidity can be a hindrance. Facilitators and program designers often need to adjust scenarios on the fly to meet learners' needs or address real-time issues.

Example: During a debriefing session, learners express confusion about the simulation objectives, prompting the need for immediate clarification or adjustments to subsequent sessions. ADDIE's linear framework doesn't always accommodate such quick pivots.

Adapting the ADDIE Model for Healthcare Simulation

To address these criticisms, healthcare simulation programs can adapt ADDIE to make it more flexible, iterative, and responsive. Below are practical strategies for modifying each phase of the model to suit the demands of healthcare education better.

1. Iterative and Agile Approaches
Instead of treating ADDIE as a strictly linear process, programs can adopt an iterative approach, allowing feedback and refinement throughout all phases.

How to Adapt:
- Treat the Evaluation phase as ongoing, incorporating formative feedback at every process stage.

- Borrow from Agile methodology by using rapid prototyping and short feedback loops.

    Example: During the Design phase of a simulation on neonatal resuscitation, pilot the initial scenario with a small group of learners. Use their feedback to refine the simulation before full-scale implementation.

2. Streamlining the Analyze Phase
The Analysis phase can be streamlined by focusing on key priorities and leveraging existing data to reduce the time and resource burden.

How to Adapt:
- Conduct a rapid needs assessment using performance data, incident reports, or surveys.

- Prioritize the most critical training needs, focusing on objectives that align with organizational goals.

    Example: Instead of conducting lengthy interviews, review error reports from the past six months to identify recurring issues, such as communication breakdowns during handoffs.

3. Modular Scenario Design
Develop modular simulations that can be quickly adapted to different contexts, reducing the time required for scenario creation.

How to Adapt:
- Create reusable components, such as standardized scripts or scenarios for common clinical situations.
- Allow facilitators to adjust complexity or focus areas based on learner needs.

Example: A cardiac arrest simulation can include optional modules, such as managing complications or incorporating family presence, to customize the experience.

4. Facilitator-Led Adaptations
Equip facilitators with tools and training to adapt simulations in real-time, addressing unexpected challenges or learner needs.

How to Adapt:
- Develop branching scenarios with multiple pathways that facilitators can activate based on learner actions.
- Train facilitators to introduce new elements or adjust pacing as needed during the simulation.

Example: In a scenario where learners miss critical patient cues, facilitators can escalate the patient's condition to refocus attention.

5. Rapid Prototyping
Incorporate rapid prototyping to test and refine scenarios early and often, ensuring that they meet learner needs without excessive delays.

How to Adapt:
- Use low-fidelity tools, such as role-playing or basic mannequins, to test scenarios before investing in high-fidelity resources.
- Conduct multiple quick iterations based on facilitator and learner feedback.

Example: A prototype simulation on infection control practices is piloted with minimal props and adjusted before full implementation.

6. Leveraging Technology
Integrate technology to streamline processes and enhance adaptability across all phases of the model.

How to Adapt:
- Use simulation software to create and modify scenarios quickly.
- Implement learning management systems (LMS) to track performance data and provide immediate feedback.

Example: A VR-based simulation allows learners to practice intubation techniques, with real-time feedback and performance metrics collected for evaluation.

Balancing Structure and Flexibility

By modifying the ADDIE model, healthcare simulation programs can retain its strengths—such as clarity, structure, and alignment—while addressing its limitations. For example:
- Using iterative feedback loops ensures continuous improvement.
- Modular and adaptable designs provide flexibility for diverse learner needs.
- Rapid prototyping and streamlined analysis enable quicker deployment without sacrificing quality.

These adaptations empower programs to meet the fast-paced, high-stakes demands of healthcare simulation while maintaining a structured approach.

Conclusion

While the ADDIE model has its critics, particularly in healthcare simulation, its principles remain valuable. By adapting the model to prioritize flexibility, rapid iteration, and real-time responsiveness, simulation programs can overcome its perceived limitations. These modifications ensure that ADDIE remains a relevant and effective framework for designing impactful training experiences, ultimately supporting improved learner performance and better patient outcomes.

Key Takeaways

1. Criticisms of ADDIE in Healthcare Simulation

- The linear and time-consuming nature of ADDIE can delay urgent training programs.
- Its perceived rigidity may limit real-time adaptability during simulations.
- ADDIE's resource-heavy demands and overemphasis on front-end analysis can be challenging for organizations with limited budgets or time constraints.

2. Adaptations for Flexibility
    - Iterative and Agile approaches can make ADDIE more dynamic, allowing for ongoing feedback and refinement throughout all phases.
    - Streamlining the Analyze phase enables quicker deployment without sacrificing relevance or effectiveness.
    - Modular scenario design and facilitator-led adaptations provide the flexibility needed to address diverse learner needs and unexpected challenges.
    - Rapid prototyping reduces development time while maintaining high-quality outcomes.
    - Leveraging technology, such as simulation software and VR, enhances adaptability and scalability across the model.

3. Balancing Structure and Adaptability
    - Modifying ADDIE to incorporate iterative feedback loops and adaptable tools ensures the model retains its structured benefits while meeting the fast-paced demands of healthcare simulation.

Reflection

The ADDIE model has been a reliable framework for instructional design for decades, providing clarity, structure, and alignment. However, its traditional approach may not always fit the high-stakes, rapidly evolving nature of healthcare simulation. Reflecting on its limitations allows us to appreciate the significance of flexibility and responsiveness in simulation-based education.

As you think about how ADDIE fits into your organization's needs, consider the following:

- Are there ways to streamline your current processes without compromising the quality of training?
- Could iterative methods or modular designs help you respond more quickly to emerging challenges?
- How can technology, such as VR or real-time analytics, support your goals?

By thoughtfully adapting ADDIE, you can create a framework that not only meets the demands of today's healthcare environment but also supports continuous improvement and innovation. This balance between structure and flexibility ensures that simulation programs remain impactful and aligned with the ultimate goal: improving learner outcomes and, ultimately, patient care.

References

Branch, R. M. (2009). *Instructional design: The ADDIE approach.* Springer Science & Business Media.

Hodell, C. (2016). *ISD: From the ground up: A concise introduction to instructional design* (4th ed.). American Society for Training and Development.

Kirkpatrick, D. L., & Kirkpatrick, J. D. (2006). *Evaluating training programs: The four levels.* Berrett-Koehler Publishers.

Morrison, G. R., Ross, S. M., Kalman, H. K., & Kemp, J. E. (2013). *Designing effective instruction* (7th ed.). Wiley.

Reigeluth, C. M. (1999). *Instructional-design theories and models: A new paradigm of instructional theory* (Vol. 2). Routledge.

Reiser, R. A., & Dempsey, J. V. (2017). *Trends and issues in instructional design and technology* (4th ed.). Pearson.

Rosen, M. A., Hunt, E. A., Pronovost, P. J., Federowicz, M. A., & Weaver, S. J. (2012). In situ simulation in continuing education for the healthcare professions: A systematic review. *Journal of Continuing Education in the Health Professions, 32*(4), 243–254. https://doi.org/10.1002/chp.21152

Zigmont, J. J., Kappus, L. J., & Sudikoff, S. N. (2011). The 3D model of debriefing: Defusing, discovering, and deepening. *Seminars in*

Perinatology, 35(2), 52–58. https://doi.org/10.1053/j.semperi.2011.01.003

"An investment in knowledge pays the best interest."
— Benjamin Franklin

Chapter 14
Quality Control in ADDIE – Ensuring Validity and Reliability of Checklists and Rubrics

Quality control is a critical component of the ADDIE model, ensuring that each phase produces outputs that align with the intended instructional goals. Nowhere is this more important than in the tools used for evaluating learner performance, such as checklists and rubrics. These tools are the foundation for assessing whether learners achieve the desired skills, knowledge, or attitudes outlined in the objectives. However, the effectiveness of these tools hinges on their validity and reliability. In healthcare simulation, where assessments often translate directly into real-world clinical practices, ensuring the quality of checklists and rubrics is not optional—it is essential.

What is Quality Control in ADDIE?

Quality control within the ADDIE framework involves continuous monitoring and refinement to ensure that the materials, processes, and outcomes meet both learner and organizational needs. For checklists and rubrics, quality control ensures that:
- The tools align closely with the learning objectives.
- They accurately measure the intended competencies.

- They produce consistent results regardless of context or evaluator.

In practice, quality control in ADDIE means revisiting and refining materials throughout the process, ensuring that each output meets high standards of educational excellence.

The Role of Validity and Reliability

Validity: Measuring the Right Things

Validity refers to the degree to which an assessment tool measures what it is intended to measure. A valid checklist or rubric in healthcare simulation accurately evaluates the critical competencies required for clinical practice. Validity ensures that learners are assessed on the skills and knowledge needed to succeed in real-world scenarios.

Why Validity Matters:
Assessment tools may evaluate irrelevant or tangential skills without validity, leaving critical competencies unmeasured.

Example: A medication administration checklist should prioritize accuracy in dosage calculation, patient identification, and timing. It lacks validity if it focuses instead on secondary skills like handwriting neatness.

Reliability: Consistent Measurement Across Contexts

Reliability refers to the consistency of an assessment tool in producing similar results across different evaluators, scenarios, or time periods. A reliable tool ensures that assessments are fair and unbiased, regardless of who conducts the evaluation or when it occurs.

Why Reliability Matters:
Inconsistent tools lead to unfair evaluations, undermining learner confidence and trust in the training program.

Example: The rubric may lack reliability if two facilitators score the same learner's CPR performance differently.

Ensuring the Validity of Checklists and Rubrics

Achieving validity involves designing tools that align directly with the instructional goals and accurately reflect the skills or knowledge being taught.

1. **Align with Learning Objectives**
   Every item on a checklist or rubric should map directly to a specific learning objective. This ensures that assessments focus on the skills learners are expected to develop.

   Example: For a trauma care scenario, the rubric should assess tasks like airway management, fluid resuscitation, and team communication, all of which are central to the learning objectives.

2. **Use Evidence-Based Criteria**
   Incorporate best practices and clinical guidelines when defining performance criteria.

   Example: A checklist for intubation might reference American Heart Association (AHA) guidelines to ensure accuracy and relevance.

3. **Consult Subject Matter Experts (SMEs)**
   Engage SMEs during the development process to verify that the assessment criteria are relevant, accurate, and comprehensive.

   Example: SMEs can confirm that a checklist for neonatal resuscitation includes essential steps like confirming proper chest rise and securing the airway.

4. **Pilot Test the Tools**
   Test the checklist or rubric with a small group of learners and facilitators to identify gaps or ambiguous criteria.

   Example: If pilot users find a rubric item unclear, such as "demonstrates effective leadership," it can be revised to specify observable behaviors like "assigns tasks clearly and confirms understanding."

5. **Eliminate Irrelevant Criteria**
   Avoid including items that do not directly contribute to evaluating the desired competencies.

   Example: A medication administration checklist should not include unrelated tasks like preparing the patient's bedside unless they are explicitly part of the objective.

Ensuring the Reliability of Checklists and Rubrics

Reliability ensures that assessments are consistent and objective, regardless of who conducts them or under what circumstances.

1. **Use Clear, Specific Language**
   Define each criterion in precise terms to minimize subjective interpretation by evaluators.

   Example: Replace "good teamwork" with "uses closed-loop communication to assign and confirm roles."

2. **Train Evaluators**
   Provide standardized training to facilitators and evaluators to ensure they apply the tools consistently.

   Example: Facilitators can practice using the rubric by scoring recorded simulation sessions and comparing their ratings.

3. **Test Inter-Rater Reliability**
   Have multiple evaluators assess the same performance and compare their scores to identify discrepancies.

   Example: If two raters differ significantly on an item, the rubric or training process may need revision.

4. **Conduct Test-Retest Reliability Checks**

Evaluate whether the tool produces consistent results when used under similar conditions at different times.

Example: If the same learner scores differently on a checklist for the same task in two identical simulations, the tool may lack reliability.

5. **Include Objective Performance Metrics**
   Where possible, incorporate objective measurements, such as time to complete a task or adherence to clinical protocols.

   Example: Use high-fidelity mannequins that track CPR metrics like depth and rate of compressions for objective scoring.

Developing High-Quality Checklists and Rubrics

To ensure both validity and reliability, follow these steps when designing checklists and rubrics:

1. **Identify Critical Competencies**
   Focus on the essential skills, knowledge, or attitudes learners must demonstrate.

   Example: A sepsis management checklist might include early recognition of symptoms, timely fluid administration, and escalation of care.

2. **Break Down Tasks**
   Divide complex tasks into smaller, measurable components.

   Example: Instead of "manage the airway," include steps like "select appropriate airway device," "position patient's head," and "confirm placement."

3. **Define Performance Levels**

Use clear, descriptive language to differentiate between levels of performance.

Example:
- *Excellent:* Administers correct dosage within 30 seconds without prompting.
- *Satisfactory:* Administers correct dosage with minor hesitation or prompting.
- *Needs Improvement:* Administers incorrect dosage or delays administration.

4. **Pilot and Refine**
Test the tools in realistic scenarios and revise based on user feedback.

Example: If facilitators find a rubric item too difficult to observe, simplify or clarify the language.

5. **Document Development and Testing**
Maintain records of how the tools were developed and tested to support ongoing quality improvement.

Example: Include SME feedback, pilot test results, and inter-rater reliability scores in your documentation.

Conclusion

Quality control in ADDIE ensures that checklists and rubrics accurately and consistently measure learner performance. By focusing on validity and reliability, healthcare simulation programs can create evaluation tools that are fair, objective, meaningful and impactful. Thoughtful development, rigorous testing, and continuous refinement of these tools ultimately contribute to better learning outcomes and improved clinical practice.

Key Takeaways

1. Validity is Critical

- Evaluation tools must measure what they are intended to measure. Valid checklists and rubrics align directly with learning objectives and focus on critical competencies.
- Using evidence-based criteria and consulting subject matter experts ensures clinical and instructional accuracy.

2. Reliability Ensures Consistency
   - Reliable tools provide consistent results across different evaluators, scenarios, and periods.
   - Clear, specific language, standardized evaluator training, and inter-rater reliability testing are essential for consistency.
3. Pilot Testing is Essential
   - Pilot testing checklists and rubrics in realistic scenarios identify gaps, ambiguities, and areas for improvement.
   - Feedback from facilitators and learners is invaluable for refining tools before full implementation.
4. Break Down Complex Tasks
   - Dividing complex skills into smaller, measurable components makes assessments more accurate and manageable.
   - For example, a task like "managing airway" can be broken down into specific, observable actions like selecting an airway device, positioning the head, and confirming placement.
5. Documentation Supports Continuous Improvement
   - Maintaining records of development and testing processes ensures transparency and supports ongoing refinement.
   - Proper documentation enables programs to track improvements and demonstrate tool effectiveness to stakeholders.

Reflection

Validity and reliability are more than technical benchmarks—they are foundational to the credibility and impact of healthcare simulation programs. A valid and reliable checklist or rubric provides clarity for learners, confidence for facilitators, and actionable insights for continuous improvement. Reflecting on your program's current practices, consider:

- **Are your evaluation tools aligned with your learning objectives?**
  Tools that stray from the intended goals risk undermining the effectiveness of the training program.
- **Do your facilitators feel confident using the evaluation tools consistently?**
  Training and practice are essential to ensure facilitators apply criteria fairly and reliably.
- **Are you using feedback to improve your tools over time?**
  A commitment to iterative refinement, informed by pilot testing and real-world feedback, strengthens the quality of your evaluation process.

By prioritizing validity, reliability, and quality control in evaluation tools, healthcare simulation programs can enhance learner outcomes and the broader impact of training initiatives, ultimately contributing to safer and more effective patient care.

References

Branch, R. M. (2009). *Instructional design: The ADDIE approach*. Springer Science & Business Media.

Gagne, R. M., Wager, W. W., Golas, K. C., & Keller, J. M. (2005). *Principles of instructional design* (5th ed.). Wadsworth/Thomson Learning.

Hodell, C. (2016). *ISD: From the ground up: A concise introduction to instructional design* (4th ed.). American Society for Training and Development.

Kirkpatrick, D. L., & Kirkpatrick, J. D. (2006). *Evaluating training programs: The four levels*. Berrett-Koehler Publishers.

Morrison, G. R., Ross, S. M., Kalman, H. K., & Kemp, J. E. (2013). *Designing effective instruction* (7th ed.). Wiley.

Reigeluth, C. M. (1999). *Instructional-design theories and models: A new paradigm of instructional theory* (Vol. 2). Routledge.

Rosen, M. A., Hunt, E. A., Pronovost, P. J., Federowicz, M. A., & Weaver, S. J. (2012). In situ simulation in continuing education for the healthcare professions: A systematic review. *Journal of*

Continuing Education in the Health Professions, 32(4), 243–254. https://doi.org/10.1002/chp.21152

Svinicki, M. D., & McKeachie, W. J. (2014). *McKeachie's teaching tips: Strategies, research, and theory for college and university teachers* (14th ed.). Wadsworth Cengage Learning.

"The purpose of learning is growth, and our minds, unlike our bodies, can continue growing as long as we live."
— Mortimer Adler

Chapter 15
The Future of ADDIE in Healthcare Simulation

The ADDIE model has been a stalwart of instructional design for decades, and its systematic approach continues to resonate in healthcare simulation. However, as healthcare faces increasingly complex challenges and educational technologies advance rapidly, ADDIE must evolve to remain relevant. This chapter envisions how ADDIE will adapt to emerging trends in simulation-based learning, exploring the integration of advanced technologies, its expansion into non-traditional applications, and how emerging instructional design methodologies can complement and enhance its structure.

As you read, imagine the possibilities of an ADDIE model that is augmented by cutting-edge technology, expands its reach into leadership and team-building simulations, and thrives in an era of iterative, learner-centered design.

Integrating Technology

Technology is reshaping every aspect of healthcare, and simulation training is no exception. By integrating technologies like virtual reality (VR), augmented reality (AR), and artificial intelligence (AI), healthcare educators can create immersive, personalized, and data-rich learning experiences. The adaptability of the ADDIE model makes it particularly well-suited for incorporating these advancements, ensuring that new tools are aligned with clear objectives and rigorous evaluation.

Virtual Reality (VR): Immersive Training Without Limits

Virtual reality creates fully immersive environments that allow learners to practice high-stakes scenarios in a safe and controlled setting. Unlike traditional simulations, VR can replicate environments and situations that may be too dangerous, rare, or costly to recreate in the real world.

Example of ADDIE Integration with VR:

- **Analysis:** Identify scenarios that require a high degree of realism or repetition, such as disaster response, neonatal resuscitation, or complex surgical procedures.
- **Design:** Collaborate with subject matter experts to design VR scenarios that replicate the sensory and procedural elements of real-world situations. Define learning objectives, such as recognizing critical signs of patient deterioration or mastering a surgical technique.
- **Development:** Partner with VR developers to create interactive, high-fidelity environments. Include branching decision pathways to simulate dynamic scenarios where learners' actions impact outcomes.
- **Implementation:** Deploy VR simulations in controlled settings, ensuring learners are oriented to the technology and provided with clear instructions. Pair VR exercises with facilitator-led debriefings to enhance learning.
- **Evaluation:** Use performance analytics from the VR platform—such as time-to-intervention or error rates—to assess learner progress. Complement this with qualitative feedback to refine the experience.

VR is particularly impactful in training for rare but critical situations, such as managing mass casualties or performing delicate neurosurgical procedures. It offers unparalleled opportunities for skill refinement, decision-making under pressure, and teamwork.

Augmented Reality (AR): Enhancing Real-World Learning

Augmented reality overlays digital information onto the physical world, enhancing traditional simulation environments with real-time, interactive data. AR applications can include step-by-step procedural guidance, anatomical overlays, or virtual patient monitors.

Example in Clinical Simulation:

In a central line placement simulation, AR could project a visual guide showing the correct insertion trajectory and real-time feedback on technique, such as depth and angle. Learners can practice more intuitively and visually richly, bridging the gap between theory and practice.

Artificial Intelligence (AI): Personalized and Scalable Learning

AI offers powerful capabilities for personalizing education, automating assessments, and scaling simulations to larger audiences. AI-powered simulations can adapt to learners' skill levels, provide tailored feedback, and analyze performance data to identify patterns and areas for improvement.

Potential AI Applications in ADDIE:

- **Analysis:** Use AI to process data from previous simulations, identifying common learner challenges and gaps in curriculum coverage.
- **Development:** Create adaptive learning pathways where the simulation adjusts difficulty based on the learner's performance.
- **Evaluation:** Employ AI-driven analytics to assess skills such as teamwork, clinical decision-making, and procedural accuracy. Intelligent algorithms can detect subtle errors or

behavioral trends, providing insights that human evaluators might miss.

By integrating these technologies, the ADDIE model can transform how simulation programs are designed, delivered, and evaluated, ensuring learners are better prepared for the complexities of modern healthcare.

Expanding ADDIE's Applications

The versatility of ADDIE extends beyond traditional clinical training. As healthcare evolves, there is a growing recognition of the need for education beyond technical skills. Leadership development, team-building, and interdisciplinary collaboration are critical for addressing the challenges of modern healthcare systems. The structured phases of ADDIE can support these broader applications, ensuring the same rigor and focus that have proven effective in clinical training.

Leadership and Team-Building Simulations

Leadership and teamwork are fundamental in healthcare, where split-second decisions and collaboration often mean the difference between life and death. Simulations designed to enhance these skills can help individuals and teams navigate challenges such as resource shortages, ethical dilemmas, or crisis management.

Example of ADDIE in Leadership Training:

- **Analysis:** Identify common leadership challenges, such as delegating tasks under pressure or managing conflict during a crisis.
- **Design:** Develop scenarios that replicate these challenges, incorporating realistic stressors such as time constraints or conflicting priorities.
- **Development:** Create interactive role-play exercises where participants rotate through leadership roles. Facilitator guides should include prompts to introduce unexpected challenges, like a sudden equipment failure or staff disagreement.

- **Implementation:** Facilitate sessions with interprofessional teams, emphasizing reflection on decision-making and team dynamics.
- **Evaluation:** Use tools like 360-degree feedback, self-assessments, and facilitator evaluations to measure outcomes.

Leadership simulations not only build individual confidence but also foster a culture of accountability and resilience across healthcare teams.

Interdisciplinary Simulations

Interdisciplinary collaboration is essential for providing holistic, patient-centered care. Simulations that bring together professionals from different disciplines can improve communication, clarify roles, and reduce errors.

Key Features of Interdisciplinary Simulations:

- **Realistic Scenarios:** Simulate complex cases, such as managing a patient with multiple comorbidities, where coordination among nurses, physicians, pharmacists, and allied health professionals is critical.
- **Role-Based Objectives:** Tailor learning objectives to each participant's role while emphasizing shared goals, such as improving patient outcomes or streamlining care transitions.
- **Debriefing Focus:** Explore how interdisciplinary teams can improve communication and address systemic barriers to collaboration.

These simulations highlight the collective strength of a well-coordinated team, preparing participants to work more effectively across disciplines.

Applications in Non-Clinical Contexts

The ADDIE model is equally applicable in non-clinical training contexts, such as public health, community outreach, and healthcare administration. For example

- **Public Health Training:** Simulate the management of a disease outbreak, training health workers to coordinate testing, treatment, and public communication.
- **Community Engagement:** Train community leaders to support vaccine campaigns or respond to natural disasters.
- **Healthcare Administration:** Develop simulations for hospital leaders to practice crisis management, resource allocation, or implementing new policies.

Trends in Instructional Design

As healthcare simulation evolves, so too does the field of instructional design. While ADDIE remains a cornerstone, new models and trends are emerging that complement and enhance its structure.

Emerging Models

1. **Agile Design:** Agile methodologies prioritize iterative development and frequent feedback. By incorporating Agile principles, ADDIE can become more dynamic and responsive to learner needs (Branch, 2009).
    - *Example:* Iteratively testing a new simulation during the Development Phase, incorporating real-time feedback from facilitators and learners.
2. **Design Thinking:** Emphasizing empathy and creativity, design thinking can enrich the Analysis and Design phases of ADDIE. By focusing deeply on learner needs, instructional designers can uncover innovative solutions.
3. **Microlearning and Gamification:** These trends address the need for flexible, engaging education. For instance, gamified simulations might include scoring systems or competitive elements to motivate learners.

Key Takeaways

1. Integrating advanced technologies like VR, AR, and AI enables the ADDIE model to deliver more immersive and personalized learning experiences.
2. ADDIE's structured approach can be adapted to broader applications, including leadership training, team-building, and interdisciplinary collaboration.
3. Emerging instructional design models, such as Agile and design thinking, complement ADDIE by fostering innovation and adaptability.
4. Trends like gamification, microlearning, and data-driven analytics are shaping the future of healthcare simulation, enhancing both learner engagement and program effectiveness.

Reflection

The future of ADDIE in healthcare simulation is brimming with potential. Consider:

- How can you leverage emerging technologies to enhance your simulation programs?
- Are there opportunities to expand ADDIE's applications in your organization, such as leadership or interdisciplinary training?
- How can you integrate trends like gamification and personalized learning into your curricula?

By embracing change and innovation, the ADDIE model will remain at the forefront of healthcare education, ensuring that simulation programs continue to inspire, challenge, and prepare healthcare professionals for the complexities of tomorrow.

Resources

Barsom, E. Z., Graafland, M., & Schijven, M. P. (2016). Systematic review on the effectiveness of augmented reality applications in medical training. *Surgical Endoscopy, 30*(10), 4174–4183. https://doi.org/10.1007/s00464-016-4800-6

Branch, R. M. (2009). *Instructional design: The ADDIE approach*. Springer Science & Business Media.

Chan, K. S., Zary, N., & Lau, Y. (2021). Artificial intelligence in medical education: A narrative review of its applications, challenges, and future perspectives. *Advances in Medical Education and Practice, 12*, 755–764. https://doi.org/10.2147/AMEP.S311054

Ellaway, R., & Topps, D. (2022). AI in healthcare education: The need for alignment with clinical priorities. *Medical Teacher, 44*(3), 229–231. https://doi.org/10.1080/0142159X.2021.2004013

Esteva, A., Robicquet, A., Ramsundar, B., Kuleshov, V., DePristo, M., Chou, K., ... & Dean, J. (2019). A guide to deep learning in healthcare. *Nature Medicine, 25*(1), 24–29. https://doi.org/10.1038/s41591-018-0316-z

Fanning, R. M., & Gaba, D. M. (2007). The role of debriefing in simulation-based learning. *Simulation in Healthcare, 2*(2), 115–125. https://doi.org/10.1097/SIH.0b013e3180315539

Gaba, D. M. (2004). The future vision of simulation in healthcare. *Quality and Safety in Health Care, 13*(Suppl 1), i2–i10. https://doi.org/10.1136/qshc.2004.009878

Holmboe, E. S., & Batalden, P. (2022). Using AI for adaptive learning in clinical education: Bridging theory and practice. *Journal of Continuing Education in the Health Professions, 42*(2), 112–118. https://doi.org/10.1097/CEH.0000000000000365

Jeffries, P. R. (2012). *Simulation in nursing education: From conceptualization to evaluation*. National League for Nursing.

Kolb, D. A. (1984). *Experiential learning: Experience as the source of learning and development*. Prentice Hall.

Kothgassner, O. D., Felnhofer, A., Hlavacs, H., Beutl, L., Palme, R., & Kryspin-Exner, I. (2012). Salivary cortisol and cardiovascular reactivity to a public speaking task in a virtual and real-life environment. *Computers in Human Behavior, 28*(2), 734–740. https://doi.org/10.1016/j.chb.2011.11.002

Kulikowski, C. A. (2019). Artificial intelligence in healthcare: Ethical considerations for the 21st century. *Artificial Intelligence in Medicine, 95*, 47–52. https://doi.org/10.1016/j.artmed.2018.11.001

Li, A., Montaño, Z., Chen, V. J., & Gold, J. I. (2011). Virtual reality and pain management: Current trends and future directions. *Pain Management, 1*(2), 147–157. https://doi.org/10.2217/pmt.10.15

Maresky, H. S., Oikonomou, A., Ali, I., Pakkal, M., Balasubramanian, A., & Bric, J. (2019). Virtual reality and cardiac anatomy: Exploring immersive three-dimensional cardiac imaging, a pilot study in undergraduate medical anatomy education. *Clinical Anatomy, 32*(2), 238–243. https://doi.org/10.1002/ca.23317

Moro, C., Štromberga, Z., Raikos, A., & Stirling, A. (2017). The effectiveness of virtual and augmented reality in health sciences and medical anatomy. *Anatomical Sciences Education, 10*(6), 549–559. https://doi.org/10.1002/ase.1696

Morrison, G. R., Ross, S. M., Kalman, H. K., & Kemp, J. E. (2013). *Designing effective instruction* (7th ed.). Wiley.

Pottle, J. (2019). Virtual reality and the transformation of medical education. *Future Healthcare Journal, 6*(3), 181–185. https://doi.org/10.7861/fhj.2019-0036

Rosen, M. A., Hunt, E. A., Pronovost, P. J., Federowicz, M. A., & Weaver, S. J. (2012). In situ simulation in continuing education for the healthcare professions: A systematic review. *Journal of Continuing Education in the Health Professions, 32*(4), 243–254. https://doi.org/10.1002/chp.21152

Schmidt, J. L., Boshuizen, H. P. A., & van Merriënboer, J. J. G. (2020). Artificial intelligence in medical education. *Medical Teacher, 42*(4), 429–434. https://doi.org/10.1080/0142159X.2019.1679638

Shaban-Nejad, A., Michalowski, M., & Buckeridge, D. L. (2018). Health intelligence: How artificial intelligence transforms personalized healthcare. *Frontiers in Artificial Intelligence, 1*, Article 1. https://doi.org/10.3389/frai.2018.00001

Sutton, R. T., Pincock, D., Baumgart, D. C., Sadowski, D. C., Fedorak, R. N., & Kroeker, K. I. (2020). An overview of clinical decision support systems: Benefits, risks, and strategies for success. *NPJ Digital Medicine, 3*, Article 17. https://doi.org/10.1038/s41746-020-0221-y

Topol, E. J. (2019). High-performance medicine: The convergence of human and artificial intelligence. *Nature Medicine, 25*(1), 44–56. https://doi.org/10.1038/s41591-018-0300-7

Zigmont, J. J., Kappus, L. J. & Sudikoff, S. N. (2011). The 3D model of debriefing: Defusing discovering, and deepening. *Seminars in Perinatology, 35*(2), 52–58. https://doi.org/10.1053/j.semperi.2011.01.003

Conclusion

Healthcare simulation stands at the intersection of education, innovation, and patient safety, playing a pivotal role in preparing healthcare professionals for the complexities of their work. The ADDIE model is central to this transformative field, a framework that brings structure, clarity, and purpose to simulation-based training. This book has explored how each phase of ADDIE—Analyze, Design, Develop, Implement, and Evaluate—is a building block for creating impactful simulations that enhance learning, improve teamwork, and ultimately contribute to better patient outcomes.

The Power of ADDIE: A Recap

The ADDIE model is not merely a process; it is a philosophy of intentionality and adaptability in instructional design. Its phased approach ensures that every step, from identifying learner needs to refining outcomes, contributes to a seamless and meaningful educational experience.

- **Analysis** ensures that training addresses specific gaps in knowledge, skills, or attitudes. By understanding the learners, their context, and organizational goals, simulation programs are tailored to meet real-world demands.

- **Design** transforms insights into actionable plans, crafting scenarios, learning objectives, and assessments that resonate with learners and reflect clinical realities.
- **Development** brings these plans to life, creating tools, environments, and materials that drive engagement and realism, whether through high-fidelity mannequins, virtual reality, or carefully scripted role-plays.
- **Implementation** turns vision into action, providing learners with immersive experiences and facilitators with clear guidance to support effective delivery.
- **Evaluation** closes the loop, offering not just a measure of success but a roadmap for improvement. It ensures that every simulation evolves to meet the changing needs of learners and the healthcare landscape.

What makes ADDIE truly powerful is its iterative nature. Each phase informs the next, creating a feedback loop that fosters continuous refinement and innovation. In an environment as dynamic as healthcare, this adaptability is critical to staying ahead of challenges and embracing opportunities.

Why Structured Instructional Design Matters

In healthcare education, the stakes are uniquely high. Success isn't simply about passing exams or mastering technical skills—it's about saving lives, improving patient outcomes, and building resilient, effective teams. In this context, adopting a structured instructional design approach like ADDIE is not just beneficial; it is essential.

Without a structured framework, simulation programs risk becoming disjointed or superficial, missing the opportunity to address deeper learning needs. ADDIE ensures that every aspect of a simulation, from the scenarios to the assessments, serves a clear and defined purpose. It bridges the gap between theory and practice, enabling learners to develop not only competence but also confidence in their abilities.

For educators and facilitators, ADDIE provides more than a roadmap—it offers a way to navigate complexity. By taking the time to analyze needs, design intentionally, and evaluate rigorously, they can create programs that are impactful, scalable, and aligned with the goals of their learners and institutions. Structured instructional design empowers educators to move beyond intuition, applying evidence-based strategies to create meaningful and lasting learning experiences.

The Role of Innovation in Shaping the Future

While ADDIE offers a solid foundation, its true potential lies in its ability to integrate new tools, technologies, and methodologies. The field of healthcare simulation is evolving rapidly, with advancements like virtual reality (VR), augmented reality (AR), and artificial intelligence (AI) transforming what is possible in education.

- **Virtual Reality** provides fully immersive environments where learners can practice high-stakes scenarios, such as disaster response or complex surgeries, without the risks of real-world consequences.
- **Augmented Reality** bridges the gap between physical and digital spaces, overlaying critical information in real time to enhance decision-making and procedural training.
- **Artificial Intelligence** enables adaptive learning, tailoring simulations to individual needs and offering data-driven insights that improve both training and assessment.

These technologies are not just innovations; they are enablers of deeper, more effective learning. When integrated into the ADDIE framework, they enhance each phase—from analyzing learner needs with AI-driven insights to developing VR scenarios that mimic real-life challenges. By embracing these tools, educators can push the boundaries of what simulation can achieve, creating programs that are as dynamic as the healthcare environment itself.

The Importance of Evaluation

Evaluation is the linchpin of the ADDIE model, ensuring that simulation programs are not static but constantly evolving. In healthcare, where best practices shift and new challenges emerge, evaluation provides the feedback necessary to keep training relevant and effective.

Through robust evaluation:

- Educators gain insight into what works and what doesn't, allowing for targeted improvements.
- Learners receive actionable feedback that helps them grow not only in skills but also in confidence.
- Organizations can measure the impact of their investment in simulation, demonstrating improvements in teamwork, safety, and patient care.

Evaluation is not the end of the process; it is the beginning of the next iteration. It is the mechanism through which programs move from good to great, and from great to transformative. By prioritizing evaluation, educators ensure that their efforts lead to meaningful change, both in the classroom and at the bedside.

Looking Ahead: A Call to Action

The future of healthcare simulation is bright, but it demands a commitment to excellence, innovation, and intentionality. As educators, facilitators, and stakeholders, we have the opportunity—and the responsibility—to shape that future by adopting frameworks like ADDIE that prioritize learner-centered design, continuous improvement, and real-world relevance.

As you reflect on the ideas and strategies presented in this book, consider:

- How can you apply the ADDIE model to address the unique challenges in your organization?
- What opportunities exist to integrate new technologies or expand your curriculum to include leadership and interdisciplinary training?
- How can you use evaluation not just as a measure of success but as a driver for innovation and growth?

DESIGN, DEVELOP, DELIVER: USING ADDIE TO BUILD EFFECTIVE HEALTHCARE SIMULATIONS

The journey to mastering healthcare simulation is ongoing, and ADDIE is your trusted guide. By applying its principles with creativity and rigor, you can create programs that inspire learners, empower teams, and, most importantly, improve patient care. Together, through thoughtful design, bold innovation, and a commitment to excellence, we can transform the future of healthcare education—one simulation at a time.

Appendices

Appendix A
Timeline of the ADDIE Model: Origins and Evolution

1940s	Programmed Instruction emerges during World War II as the U.S. military develops systematic training approaches to train large numbers of personnel efficiently.
1950s	Early systems-based instructional design approaches are formalized, emphasizing breaking tasks into smaller units and aligning instruction with measurable goals.
1960s	- Robert Gagné introduces Nine Events of Instruction, focusing on structured instructional sequences. - Bloom's Taxonomy provides a framework for defining clear learning objectives.
1970s	- The ADDIE model is formally developed by the Center for Educational Technology at Florida State University for the U.S. Army to standardize training design through the Instructional Systems Design (ISD) process. - Emphasis on the phased approach (Analyze, Design, Develop, Implement, Evaluate) for systematic alignment.
1980s	ADDIE gains widespread adoption in corporate training and higher education, becoming a standard framework for developing scalable, efficient training programs.
1990s	Refinements to ADDIE emerge: - Gagné's Conditions of Learning integrate further with the model. - Critiques arise about its perceived rigidity and sequential nature, prompting iterative modifications.
2000s	ADDIE adapts to the rise of e-learning and digital training platforms, incorporating new technologies like Learning Management Systems (LMS). Emphasis shifts to learner-centered design.
2010s	ADDIE is blended with Agile methodologies to create iterative, flexible processes. The rise of virtual reality (VR) and augmented reality (AR) influences the Develop and Implement phases.
2020s–Present	- Incorporation of Artificial Intelligence (AI) and adaptive learning technologies into the Develop and Evaluate phases. - ADDIE is integrated with microlearning, gamification, and data-driven analytics for personalized and engaging educational experiences.

Appendix B
Sample Scenarios

Managing a Patient with Sepsis

Note: This sample represents the steps in the ADDIE Process. The actual length and number of documents will vary based on the scenario and the training needs.

1. Analyze

Goal:
Train healthcare providers to promptly identify and manage sepsis using evidence-based guidelines, ultimately reducing time-to-treatment and improving patient outcomes.

Needs Assessment:
Sepsis is a leading cause of mortality, with delays in diagnosis and treatment being major contributors to poor outcomes (Singer et al., 2016). A review of internal performance data shows variability in recognizing early sepsis indicators and initiating treatment. Simulation training is needed to provide hands-on experience with high-risk scenarios.

Target Audience:

- **Primary Learners:** Nurses and physicians working in emergency or critical care.
- **Skill Level:** Intermediate to advanced clinicians familiar with sepsis guidelines but needing practice in rapid recognition and team-based intervention.

Objectives:
By the end of the simulation learners will:

1. **Identify:** Early warning signs of sepsis using Sepsis-3 criteria.
2. **Prioritize:** Initiate fluid resuscitation, obtain cultures, and administer antibiotics within 60 minutes.
3. **Communicate:** Use structured SBAR communication to escalate care to ICU or other advanced levels.

Deliverables:

- Needs analysis report detailing gaps in current practice.
- Learning objectives aligned with Sepsis-3 criteria and institutional goals.
- Defined target audience and stakeholder list (clinical educators, nurse managers, simulation staff).

---

2. Design

Scenario Overview:
This scenario replicates an emergency department setting where a patient presents with signs of sepsis. The focus is on clinical decision-making, adherence to protocols, and team communication under time pressure.

Learning Objectives:

1. Recognize clinical indicators of sepsis: altered mental status, hypotension, elevated heart rate, tachypnea, and fever.
2. Administer a 30 mL/kg fluid bolus and prescribe broad-spectrum antibiotics per protocol.
3. Ensure clear, concise communication during care escalation.

Key Scenario Details:

- **Patient Profile:**
    - 68-year-old male presenting with fever, confusion, hypotension, and recent history of a urinary tract infection.

        - Vital Signs: HR 120 bpm, RR 28/min, BP 88/50, Temp 39.2°C, SpO2 91%.
        - Labs: Elevated lactate (4.8 mmol/L), WBC 18,000, creatinine 2.0 mg/dL.
- **Setting:** Emergency department resuscitation room with bedside monitors and supplies.
- **Learner Roles:**
    - Primary RN: Assessment and IV administration.
    - MD: Decision-making (diagnosis, orders for labs and treatments).
    - Secondary RN: Assisting with fluid and medication preparation.

Assessment Metrics:

- Time-to-antibiotics administration.
- Accurate application of the "Sepsis Bundle."
- Communication effectiveness during SBAR reports.

Deliverables:

- Scenario script detailing patient presentation, clinical progression, and expected learner actions.
- Learner roles and responsibilities guide.
- Assessment rubrics to track performance during the simulation.
- Scenario briefing and debriefing templates.

---

3. Develop

Simulation Materials:

- **Patient Details:**
    - A pre-programmed high-fidelity manikin that can mimic altered mental status, tachypnea, hypotension, and responses to treatment.
- **Scenario Programming:**

- Realistic vital sign changes: BP and SpO2 drop if interventions are delayed, and lactate normalizes after treatment.
- **Pre-Simulation Materials:**
  - **Handouts:** Summary of Sepsis-3 criteria and treatment protocols.
  - **Infographics:** Visual flowcharts of the Sepsis Bundle for quick reference.
  - **Video Resource:** Example of SBAR communication for care escalation.
- **Facilitator Training Package:**
  - Instructional guides on how to run the simulation, manage manikin responses, and facilitate the debrief session.
  - Checklist for facilitators to track learners' actions in real-time.

Additional Development Deliverables:

- Fully programmed simulation scenario on a high-fidelity simulator.
- Pre-simulation orientation materials for learners and facilitators.
- Customized environment setup, including patient monitors, medications (mock saline, antibiotics), and lab results.

---

4. Implement

Simulation Schedule:
The session is designed for small groups of 3–5 participants, allowing everyone to play an active role. Each session lasts 50 minutes (5-minute pre-brief, 30-minute scenario, 15-minute debrief).

Session Plan:

1. **Pre-Brief (5 minutes):**

- Introduce objectives, environment, and expectations.
- Familiarize learners with the equipment and simulation rules.
2. **Scenario Execution (30 minutes):**
    - Patient presents with altered mental status, hypotension, and fever.
    - Learners must assess the patient, interpret lab results, and initiate treatment.
    - If no interventions occur within 10 minutes, the patient deteriorates, developing septic shock.
3. **Debrief (15 minutes):**
    - Review clinical decisions and teamwork.
    - Connect actions to patient outcomes using facilitator-led discussion.

Staff Training:

Before launching the simulation, facilitators undergo training sessions to:

- Operate the simulation equipment.
- Follow the scenario script.
- Facilitate effective debrief sessions.

Deliverables:

- Session schedules with learner assignments.
- Pre-briefing and debriefing materials for facilitators.
- Facilitator training guides.

---

5. Evaluate

Formative Evaluation:

- **During Simulation:** Facilitators use a structured checklist to assess whether learners recognize sepsis, initiate appropriate interventions, and communicate effectively.

Summative Evaluation:

- **Post-Simulation Assessment:** A written test or Objective Structured Clinical Examination (OSCE) to evaluate knowledge retention and application.

Learner Feedback:

- Participants complete surveys rating scenario realism, difficulty, and impact on their clinical confidence.

Outcome Evaluation:

- Measure clinical performance metrics (e.g., time to antibiotic administration) in real patient care settings 3–6 months after training.

Deliverables:

- Learner performance data (checklists, tests).
- Participant feedback survey results.
- Summary report of simulation outcomes, including recommendations for scenario improvements.

Key Deliverables Overview

1. **Analyze:** Needs assessment report, learner objectives, and target audience profile.
2. **Design:** Scenario script, learner role descriptions, and assessment rubrics.
3. **Develop:** Pre-simulation resources (handouts, infographics, videos), programmed simulation software, and facilitator guides.
4. **Implement:** Session schedules, facilitator training materials, and pre-brief/debrief resources.

5. **Evaluate:** Learner assessment data, participant feedback surveys, and an outcome evaluation report.

Breaking Bad News to a Patient and Family

Note: This sample represents the steps in the ADDIE Process. The actual length and number of documents will vary based on the scenario and the training needs.

1. Analyze

Goal:
Equip healthcare professionals with the communication skills needed to deliver bad news empathetically, clearly, and effectively, while addressing emotional responses and fostering trust.

Needs Assessment:
Research indicates that many healthcare professionals struggle with delivering bad news due to a lack of formal training, leading to patient dissatisfaction and increased stress for clinicians (Baile et al., 2000). Simulation-based learning is ideal for providing practice in a controlled, reflective environment.

Target Audience:

- **Primary Learners:** Physicians, nurse practitioners, and advanced practice providers in oncology, palliative care, or critical care settings.
- **Skill Level:** Intermediate learners with basic knowledge of patient-centered communication but limited experience delivering bad news in real-world scenarios.

Objectives:
By the end of the simulation, learners will:

1. Utilize a structured framework (e.g., SPIKES) for breaking bad news.

2. Demonstrate empathy and active listening while addressing emotional responses.
3. Provide clear, concise, and honest information about the prognosis or diagnosis.
4. Collaborate with the patient and/or family to discuss next steps and support options.

Deliverables:

- Needs analysis report summarizing gaps in communication skills.
- Defined learning objectives aligned with professional standards for empathetic communication.
- Audience profile and list of key stakeholders (clinical educators, simulation staff).

---

2. Design

Scenario Overview:
This simulation recreates a clinical consultation where the learner must deliver a life-changing diagnosis (e.g., metastatic cancer) to a patient and their family member.

Learning Objectives:

1. Apply the SPIKES protocol (Setting, Perception, Invitation, Knowledge, Emotions, Summary) or a similar structured communication model.
2. Balance medical accuracy with compassionate communication.
3. Offer emotional support and respond to patient/family questions effectively.

Key Scenario Details:

- **Patient Profile:**

- o 52-year-old female patient recently diagnosed with metastatic lung cancer.
- o Family member (daughter, 28 years old) accompanies the patient.
- **Setting:** Oncology consultation room equipped with chairs, tissues, and educational materials.
- **Learner Roles:**
  - o Primary provider: Delivers the news and facilitates discussion.
  - o Observer(s): Peers or facilitators who provide feedback post-simulation.

Assessment Metrics:

- Adherence to the SPIKES protocol.
- Demonstrated empathy through verbal and non-verbal communication.
- Clarity and accuracy of the information shared.
- Ability to manage emotional responses effectively.

Deliverables:

- Scenario script detailing patient and family reactions, including emotional cues and potential questions.
- Learner role descriptions and facilitator guide.
- Rubric for assessing communication performance.

---

3. Develop

Simulation Materials:

- **Role-Playing Characters:**
  - o Patient actor (standardized patient): Nervous and fearful but composed.
  - o Family member actor: Initially calm but becomes emotional upon hearing the news.
- **Pre-Simulation Resources:**

- - **Handouts:** Summary of the SPIKES protocol and best practices for delivering bad news.
    - **Video Resource:** Example of a clinician delivering bad news empathetically.
    - **Checklist:** Key phrases and behaviors to use or avoid during the conversation.
- **Room Setup:**
    - Comfortable, private consultation room with seating arranged to promote eye contact.
    - Props: Tissues, patient medical chart, and educational brochures on palliative care or treatment options.

Scripts and Prompts:

- Patient: "I've been worried about this for weeks. Can you just tell me what's going on?"
- Family Member: "What does this mean for her? Are you saying there's nothing we can do?"
- **Learner Prompts:**
    - Facilitator ensures learners stay on track if they struggle (e.g., "What might be a helpful way to respond to the family member's emotions?").

Additional Development Deliverables:

- Fully scripted scenario for standardized patients, including potential patient/family responses to learner actions.
- Pre-simulation orientation guide for participants.
- Emotional debriefing framework for facilitators to support learners after the session.

---

4. Implement

Simulation Schedule:

- Sessions designed for small groups (3–4 participants) to maximize individual feedback. Each session lasts 50 minutes (5-minute pre-brief, 30-minute scenario, 15-minute debrief).

Session Plan:

1. **Pre-Brief (5 minutes):**
   - Explain simulation objectives, introduce the SPIKES framework, and set expectations for professionalism.
   - Review the importance of self-reflection and peer feedback.
2. **Scenario Execution (30 minutes):**
   - Patient and family actors engage in the scripted consultation.
   - Learner must navigate breaking bad news, addressing emotional reactions, and collaborating on a care plan.
3. **Debrief (15 minutes):**
   - Facilitator-led discussion focusing on what went well, what could be improved, and how learners felt during the interaction.
   - Provide feedback on empathy, clarity, and adherence to the SPIKES protocol.

Staff Training:
Facilitators and standardized patients undergo training to:

- Follow the scripted scenario while allowing flexibility for learner responses.
- Deliver constructive feedback during debrief sessions.
- Recognize and manage learner stress or emotional responses.

Deliverables:

- Session schedules with learner assignments.
- Pre-briefing and debriefing materials for facilitators.
- Training materials for standardized patients and facilitators.

5. Evaluate

Formative Evaluation:

- **During Simulation:** Facilitators use a checklist to assess learner performance on key communication skills (e.g., empathy, clarity, responsiveness).
- Peer observers provide additional feedback.

Summative Evaluation:

- **Post-Simulation Assessment:** Learners complete a reflective self-assessment and a short multiple-choice test on the SPIKES protocol.

Learner Feedback:

- Participants complete surveys to evaluate the simulation's realism, relevance, and impact on their confidence.

Outcome Evaluation:

- Conduct follow-up evaluations (e.g., direct observation or patient satisfaction surveys) in clinical practice to assess the application of skills learned.

Deliverables:

- Learner performance data, including completed checklists and test scores.
- Feedback survey results summarizing learner experience and suggestions for improvement.
- Post-simulation outcome evaluation report.

Key Deliverables Overview

1. **Analyze:** Needs analysis report, learning objectives, and audience profile.
2. **Design:** Scenario script, learner roles, and assessment rubric.
3. **Develop:** Pre-simulation resources (handouts, videos, checklists), scripts for standardized patients, and facilitator guides.
4. **Implement:** Session schedules, standardized patient training materials, and debriefing resources.
5. **Evaluate:** Learner assessments, feedback surveys, and outcome evaluation report.

Urosepsis vs. Malignant Hypothermia

Note: This sample represents the steps in the ADDIE Process. The actual length and number of documents will vary based on the scenario and the training needs.

1. Analyze

Goal:
Train healthcare providers to distinguish between two critical conditions—urosepsis and malignant hyperthermia (MH)—based on clinical presentation and implement appropriate interventions.

Needs Assessment:
Misdiagnosis or delayed diagnosis of urosepsis or MH can lead to rapid patient deterioration and mortality. A review of clinical errors in acute care settings reveals challenges in differentiating between systemic infections and rare but life-threatening complications like MH, particularly in perioperative environments.

Target Audience:
- **Primary Learners:** Physicians, nurse practitioners, anesthesiologists, critical care nurses, and OR staff.

- **Skill Level:** Intermediate-to-advanced clinicians familiar with basic sepsis and MH criteria but needing improved diagnostic reasoning and hands-on experience.

Objectives:
By the end of the simulation, learners will:

1. Differentiate urosepsis and malignant hyperthermia based on clinical presentation and history.
2. Prioritize interventions tailored to the specific condition (e.g., broad-spectrum antibiotics for urosepsis or dantrolene administration for MH).
3. Communicate effectively with interdisciplinary teams to escalate care.

Deliverables:

- Needs analysis report summarizing diagnostic challenges.
- Learning objectives aligned with diagnostic criteria for urosepsis and MH.
- Audience profile and list of stakeholders (clinical educators, simulation staff, anesthesiology leadership).

---

2. Design

Scenario Overview:
This simulation challenges learners to assess and manage a patient presenting with overlapping signs of both conditions (e.g., fever, tachycardia, muscle rigidity). The scenario unfolds in two possible pathways: urosepsis or malignant hyperthermia, depending on the learner's decisions and interventions.

Learning Objectives:

1. Accurately interpret clinical data to differentiate between urosepsis and MH.

2. Initiate appropriate interventions for the identified condition within 15 minutes.
3. Collaborate with the care team to stabilize the patient.

Key Scenario Details:

- **Patient Profile:**
    - 45-year-old male who recently underwent abdominal surgery under general anesthesia.
    - Presents with fever, tachycardia, and muscle rigidity in the post-anesthesia care unit (PACU).
- **Setting:** PACU or ICU equipped with monitoring equipment and emergency supplies.
- **Scenario Pathways:**
    - **Urosepsis Pathway:** Patient recently discharged from the hospital for a urinary tract infection. Vital signs indicate hypotension, fever, and altered mental status.
    - **Malignant Hyperthermia Pathway:** Recent surgery under general anesthesia, presenting with hypercapnia (increased $EtCO_2$), muscle rigidity, and hyperthermia.

Assessment Metrics:

- Ability to identify the correct condition based on key indicators (e.g., history of recent UTI vs. anesthetic exposure).
- Timely initiation of appropriate interventions.
- Effective team communication and escalation of care.

Deliverables:

- Scenario script detailing clinical presentation and potential learner decisions.
- Learner role descriptions and facilitator guides.
- Assessment rubric for evaluating clinical reasoning, timeliness of interventions, and communication.

3. Develop

Simulation Materials:

- **Patient Data:**
    - **Urosepsis:** Elevated lactate (4.5 mmol/L), WBC 18,000, creatinine 2.2 mg/dL, low BP (88/50 mmHg), and fever (39.5°C).
    - **MH:** Rapidly rising EtCO2, hyperthermia (40.5°C), muscle rigidity, tachycardia (140 bpm), and metabolic acidosis.
- **Manikin Programming:**
    - Pathway-specific changes in vital signs based on learner interventions.
    - Deterioration if appropriate interventions are delayed (e.g., sepsis progressing to septic shock, MH leading to cardiac arrest).
- **Pre-Simulation Resources:**
    - **Handouts:** Diagnostic criteria for urosepsis (Sepsis-3 guidelines) and MH (MHAUS protocols).
    - **Flowcharts:** Side-by-side comparison of clinical signs and treatments.
    - **Video Resource:** Demonstration of dantrolene preparation and administration.
- **Equipment and Props:**
    - **For Urosepsis Pathway:** IV antibiotics (mock medications), fluid resuscitation supplies, and Foley catheter.
    - **For MH Pathway:** Dantrolene, cooling blankets, and an arterial blood gas (ABG) analysis machine.
- **Facilitator Prompts:**
    - "The patient's EtCO2 is rising rapidly." (MH cue)
    - "The patient's BP is dropping despite fluid administration." (Urosepsis cue)

Additional Development Deliverables:

- Fully programmed manikin scenarios for both urosepsis and MH pathways.
- Pre-simulation orientation materials for learners.
- Facilitator and standardized patient training guides.

4. Implement

Simulation Schedule:
Small-group sessions (3–5 participants per session) to promote active participation and team-based learning. Each session lasts 50 minutes (5-minute pre-brief, 30-minute scenario, 15-minute debrief).

Session Plan:

1. **Pre-Brief (5 minutes):**
   - Review objectives, simulation environment, and roles.
   - Highlight the importance of differentiating between overlapping conditions.
2. **Scenario Execution (30 minutes):**
   - Patient presents in PACU with fever, tachycardia, and muscle rigidity.
   - Learners gather history, interpret clinical data, and decide on interventions.
   - Depending on actions, the scenario proceeds toward either urosepsis (e.g., fluid resuscitation and antibiotics) or MH (e.g., dantrolene and cooling).
3. **Debrief (15 minutes):**
   - Facilitator-led discussion on clinical reasoning, teamwork, and management decisions.
   - Highlight key differences in presentation and treatment between the two conditions.

Staff Training:
Facilitators and standardized patients are trained to:

- Monitor learner performance and provide subtle cues if learners struggle.

- Conduct debriefs using structured reflection models (e.g., PLUS/DELTA).

Deliverables:

- Session schedules with learner roles and assignments.
- Pre-brief and debrief templates.
- Training materials for facilitators and actors.

---

5. Evaluate

Formative Evaluation:

- **During Simulation:** Facilitators use a checklist to assess learner decisions, including diagnosis accuracy, intervention timing, and communication.
- Peer observers provide feedback on teamwork and clinical reasoning.

Summative Evaluation:

- **Post-Simulation Test:** Learners complete a short quiz on key diagnostic and treatment differences between urosepsis and MH.

Learner Feedback:

- Surveys assess the simulation's realism, complexity, and value for clinical practice.

Outcome Evaluation:

- Measure clinical performance outcomes (e.g., time-to-diagnosis or treatment) in simulated and real-world settings.

Deliverables:

- Learner performance data (checklists, quiz scores).
- Feedback surveys summarizing learner experience.
- Post-simulation evaluation report, including recommendations for scenario improvements.

Key Deliverables Overview

1. **Analyze:** Needs analysis report, learning objectives, and audience profile.
2. **Design:** Scenario script, learner roles, assessment rubrics, and clinical pathways.
3. **Develop:** Pre-simulation resources (handouts, videos, flowcharts), manikin programming, and facilitator guides.
4. **Implement:** Session schedules, pre-briefing materials, and facilitator training resources.
5. **Evaluate:** Learner assessments, feedback surveys, and post-simulation evaluation report.

Appendix C
Templates for ADDIE Phases

Below are sample templates for each phase of the ADDIE model, designed to be adaptable to various healthcare simulation contexts.

1. Analysis Phase Template

Purpose: To gather information about learner needs, organizational goals, and training requirements.

Analysis Report Template

Section	Details
Project Title:	Name of the simulation project or curriculum.
Date:	Date of the analysis report.
Prepared By:	Name(s) of the individual(s) conducting the analysis.
Target Audience:	- Who are the learners? - What are their roles and experience levels?
Learning Needs:	- What gaps in knowledge, skills, or attitudes exist?
Organizational Goals:	- What are the broader goals of the organization or department?
Desired Outcomes:	- What measurable outcomes should result from the training?
Constraints:	- Budget, time, resources, or other limitations.
Data Collection Methods:	- Surveys, interviews, focus groups, incident reports, etc.
Key Findings:	- Summary of the most critical insights from the analysis.

2. Design Phase Template

Purpose: To translate the findings from the analysis phase into a detailed simulation plan.

Scenario Design Document

Section	Details
Scenario Title:	Name of the scenario (e.g., "Sepsis Management in the ICU").
Rationale:	- List specific rationale for the scenario/educational activity
Learning Objectives:	- List specific, measurable objectives (e.g., "Demonstrate early recognition of sepsis").
Target Audience:	- Who will participate? Include roles (e.g., nurses, physicians).
Learner/facilitator Prerequisites:	- List any learner prerequisites - List any facilitator prerequisites
Scenario Description:	- Brief overview of the scenario's clinical context.
Clinical Setting:	- ICU, ER, community health clinic, etc.
Scenario Flow:	- **Stage 1:** Initial patient presentation. - **Stage 2:** Clinical triggers/events. - **Stage 3:** Resolution or escalation.
Roles and Responsibilities:	- Role of each participant (e.g., team leader, bedside nurse, family member).
Equipment/Resources Needed:	- Mannequins, monitors, props, patient charts, etc.
Critical Events:	- Specific events or conditions to trigger during the scenario.
Facilitator Guide:	- Detailed instructions for facilitators, including prompts and cues.
Assessment Criteria:	- List key behaviors to observe, aligned with learning objectives.

3. Development Phase Template

Purpose: To create the tools, resources, and materials needed for the simulation.

Resource Development Checklist

Resource	Details
Scenario Script:	Detailed dialogue and events for facilitators and actors (if applicable).
Lesson Plan:	As applicable
Role Descriptions:	Clear guidelines for each participant role.

DESIGN, DEVELOP, DELIVER: USING ADDIE TO BUILD EFFECTIVE HEALTHCARE SIMULATIONS

Resource	Details
Facilitator Guide:	Step-by-step instructions, debriefing prompts, and troubleshooting tips.
Simulation Environment Setup:	List of required equipment, props, and environment details.
Learner Materials:	Pre-simulation readings, checklists, job aids, or procedural guides.
Assessment Tools:	Rubrics, observation checklists, or scoring sheets.
Technology Requirements:	Description of VR/AR systems, AI tools, or simulation software needed.

4. Implementation Phase Template

Purpose: To organize the logistics and ensure smooth delivery of the simulation.

Implementation Plan

Section	Details
Session Schedule:	- Dates, times, and durations for each session.
Participant Preparation:	- Pre-simulation materials provided (e.g., guidelines, videos).
Facilitator Roles:	- Specific tasks for each facilitator during the simulation.
Environment Setup:	- Step-by-step checklist for setting up the simulation environment.
Equipment Testing:	- Procedures to ensure all technology and equipment are functioning properly.
Contingency Plans:	- Backup plans for technical issues, participant absences, or other disruptions.
Session Agenda:	- Detailed timeline, including pre-briefing, simulation, and debriefing activities.

5. Evaluation Phase Template

Purpose: To assess the effectiveness of the simulation and identify areas for improvement.

Evaluation Form

Section	Details
Simulation Title:	Name of the scenario or training session.
Date:	Date of the simulation.
Evaluator Name:	Name(s) of the evaluator(s).
Assessment Criteria:	- List specific behaviors/skills to evaluate, aligned with objectives.
Learner Feedback:	- **What did you find most valuable about the simulation?** - **Were the objectives clear?** - **How realistic was the scenario?**
Facilitator Feedback:	- Did the scenario flow as expected? - Were any adjustments needed during delivery?
Performance Metrics:	- Quantitative measures (e.g., time-to-intervention, error rates).
Overall Effectiveness:	- Summary of whether objectives were met and key outcomes achieved.
Recommendations:	- Suggestions for improvement or refinement of the simulation.

Appendix C
ADDIE Inputs and Outputs

Analysis Phase	
Inputs	**Outputs (Deliverables)**
☐ Organizational Need ☐ Stakeholder Input ☐ Job & Task Analysis ☐ Learner Demographics & Characteristics ☐ Data Collection Methods ☐ Constraints & Resources	☐ Defined Learning Needs ☐ Target Audience Profile ☐ Learning Objectives ☐ Scope of Training ☐ Data-driven Insights ☐ Constraints & Assumptions ☐ Analysis Report

Design Phase	
Inputs	**Outputs (Deliverables)**
☐ Defined Learning Needs ☐ Target Audience Profile ☐ Learning Objectives ☐ Scope of Training ☐ Data-driven Insights ☐ Constraints & Assumptions ☐ Analysis Report	☐ Detailed Learning Objectives ☐ Scenario Plans ☐ Assessment Tools ☐ Instructional Strategies ☐ Pre-simulation Materials ☐ Facilitator Guides ☐ Storyboards/flowcharts ☐ Evaluation Plan

Development Phase

Inputs	Outputs (Deliverables)
☐ Detailed Learning Objectives ☐ Scenario Plans ☐ Assessment Tools ☐ Instructional Strategies ☐ Pre-simulation Materials ☐ Facilitator Guides ☐ Storyboards/flowcharts ☐ Evaluation Plan	☐ Simulation Scenarios & Scripts ☐ Instructional Materials ☐ Assessment Tools ☐ Facilitator Resources ☐ Simulation Environment Setup ☐ Technology & Media Development ☐ Tested Materials ☐ Revised & Finalized Content

Implementation Phase

Inputs	Outputs (Deliverables)
☐ Simulation Scenarios & Scripts ☐ Instructional Materials ☐ Assessment Tools ☐ Facilitator Resources ☐ Simulation Environment Setup ☐ Technology & Media Development ☐ Tested Materials ☐ Revised & Finalized Content	☐ Delivered Simulation Sessions ☐ Learner Engagement & Participation ☐ Facilitator Performance ☐ Performance Data Collection ☐ Formative Feedback for Learners ☐ Debriefing Sessions ☐ Identified Challenges or Gaps ☐ Feedback from Participants

Evaluation Phase	
Inputs	**Outputs (Deliverables)**
☐ Learning Objectives ☐ Assessment Tools ☐ Performance Data ☐ Learner Feedback ☐ Facilitator Feedback ☐ Simulation Observations ☐ Organizational Goals & Metrics	☐ Evaluation Report ☐ Performance Metrics ☐ Participant Feedback Summary ☐ Facilitator Feedback Summary ☐ Recommendations for Refinement ☐ Actionable Changes for Future Interventions ☐ Organizational Impact Data ☐ Iterative Design Plan

This table reflects the structured nature of the ADDIE model, ensuring that each phase flows logically into the next.

Each phase of the ADDIE model is deeply interconnected. For example, the outputs of the Analyze phase serve as inputs for the Design phase, creating a seamless flow. By maintaining a structured yet flexible approach, the ADDIE model helps ensure instructional programs are effective and aligned with learner needs and organizational goals.

KEITH A. BEAULIEU

Appendix D
ADDIE Model Checklist

1. Analysis Phase Checklist

- ☐ Define the problem or gap in knowledge, skills, or attitudes.
- ☐ Identify the target audience, including demographics and experience levels.
- ☐ Gather data through:
  - o Surveys
  - o Interviews
  - o Focus groups
  - o Incident reports
- ☐ Outline specific organizational goals for the training program.
- ☐ Establish desired outcomes that are measurable and realistic.
- ☐ Assess available resources (e.g., budget, technology, time).
- ☐ Identify potential constraints or challenges.
- ☐ Summarize findings in an analysis report.

2. Design Phase Checklist

- ☐ Develop clear, measurable learning objectives.
- ☐ Create a high-level outline of the simulation curriculum.
- ☐ Map learning objectives to specific scenarios or activities.
- ☐ Incorporate relevant learning theories (e.g., adult learning principles, experiential learning).
- ☐ Design realistic and evidence-based scenarios:
  - o Define the clinical context.
  - o Specify roles for participants.
  - o Include key events or triggers.
- ☐ Plan debriefing and feedback strategies.
- ☐ Determine assessment tools and methods:
  - o Rubrics
  - o Checklists
  - o Observation forms
- ☐ Draft facilitator guides and learner materials.

3. Development Phase Checklist

- ☐ Develop detailed scenario scripts and flowcharts.
- ☐ Prepare facilitator guides with:
    - Instructions
    - Prompts
    - Troubleshooting tips
- ☐ Create or gather necessary resources:
    - Mannequins
    - Equipment
    - Props
    - Technology (e.g., VR/AR systems)
- ☐ Test all equipment and technology to ensure functionality.
- ☐ Develop pre-simulation learner materials (e.g., guidelines, case studies).
- ☐ Create assessment tools (e.g., rubrics, scoring sheets).
- ☐ Conduct pilot testing to:
    - Validate scenario flow.
    - Identify and address gaps or challenges.
    - Collect feedback from test participants and facilitators.

4. Implementation Phase Checklist

- ☐ Schedule simulation sessions and confirm availability of all participants and facilitators.
- ☐ Distribute pre-simulation materials to learners.
- ☐ Prepare the simulation environment:
    - Set up equipment and props.
    - Arrange the space to reflect the clinical setting.
    - Test technology (e.g., monitors, VR systems).
- ☐ Brief facilitators on:
    - Learning objectives
    - Scenario flow
    - Assessment methods
- ☐ Conduct a pre-briefing session with learners:
    - Introduce objectives and structure.
    - Establish psychological safety.
- ☐ Facilitate the simulation, ensuring:
    - Realism and engagement.
    - Smooth scenario progression.
- ☐ Address challenges or deviations in real-time.
- ☐ Conduct a structured debriefing session after each simulation.

DESIGN, DEVELOP, DELIVER: USING ADDIE TO BUILD EFFECTIVE
HEALTHCARE SIMULATIONS

5. Evaluation Phase Checklist

- [ ] Collect feedback from learners through:
    - Surveys
    - Self-assessments
    - Focus groups
- [ ] Gather feedback from facilitators on:
    - Scenario flow and realism.
    - Challenges encountered.
- [ ] Analyze performance data using:
    - Rubrics
    - Observation checklists
    - Technology-generated metrics (e.g., VR/AR performance data).
- [ ] Compare outcomes to learning objectives to measure success.
- [ ] Identify trends or common gaps in learner performance.
- [ ] Compile findings into an evaluation report.
- [ ] Use feedback to refine the simulation:
    - Adjust scenarios, resources, or assessments.
    - Update facilitator guides or learner materials.
- [ ] Share results with stakeholders to demonstrate program impact.

KEITH A. BEAULIEU

Appendix E
ADDIE Deliverable Checklist

1. Analyze Phase

- ☐ **Needs Assessment Document(s)**
    - Clear identification of the performance gap or problem
    - Description of target audience demographics, skills, and preferences
    - Stakeholder interviews or focus group summaries
    - Current process or workflow documentation

- ☐ **Goal Alignment Document(s)**
    - Defined project goals and objectives
    - Alignment with organizational mission or goals

- ☐ **Resource Identification Document(s)**
    - Available tools, technologies, and budget
    - Potential constraints or risks identified

- ☐ **Gap Analysis Report**
    - Summary of current vs. desired performance
    - Recommendations for addressing gaps

2. Design Phase

- ☐ **Learning Objectives Document(s)**

- Clear, measurable, and aligned objectives (using Bloom's Taxonomy)
- Alignment of objectives with the target audience needs

☐ **Instructional Strategies Document(s)**

- Outlined teaching methods (e.g., scenario-based learning, e-learning, etc.)
- Proposed assessment strategies

☐ **Content Outline**

- Detailed module or lesson breakdown
- Storyboards or wireframes (for e-learning or media)

☐ **Design Documents**

- Initial prototypes or mockups
- Documentation of chosen technology/tools

☐ **Approval Milestones**

- Stakeholder sign-off on design documents

3. Develop Phase

☐ **Content Development Document(s)**

- Creation of learning materials (e.g., presentations, e-learning modules, videos, etc.)
- Scripts for media components
- Printable job aids, guides, or handouts

☐ **Technology Integration**

- o Development of LMS components (if applicable)
- o Testing of technical elements (e.g., SCORM packages, simulations, interactive elements)

☐ **Review and Iteration Document(s)**

- o Internal quality assurance checks
- o Stakeholder review and feedback loop

☐ **Finalized Deliverables**

- o <u>Completed course materials</u>
- o Documentation of technical setup/integration

---

4. Implement Phase

☐ **Training Setup Document(s)**

- o Installation and configuration of LMS, software, or tools
- o Venue or virtual platform readiness (if live training)

☐ **Facilitator Preparation Document(s)**

- o Training guides for instructors or facilitators
- o Pre-training briefings or workshops

☐ **Pilot Testing**

- o Conduct of pilot sessions
- o Feedback collection from pilot participants

☐ **Delivery**

- o Smooth rollout of training to target audience

- Attendance tracking and engagement monitoring

5. Evaluate Phase

- **Formative Evaluation Document(s)**
    - Ongoing feedback during each phase
    - Documentation of challenges and adjustments

- **Summative Evaluation Document(s)**
    - Collection of post-training feedback (e.g., surveys, interviews, assessments)
    - Assessment of learner performance vs. objectives

- **Impact Analysis Document(s)**
    - Measurable impact on performance gaps (KPIs, ROI, etc.)
    - Stakeholder review of results

- **Additional Organizational Data Documents(s)**
    - Additional data that may come in during the lifecycle of the training that may affect the lessons learned and recommendations.

- **Final Report**
    - Comprehensive summary of project outcomes
    - Lessons learned and recommendations for future projects

Note: Many organizations will want a comprehensive report, a succinct summary, and a PowerPoint presentation/slide deck. Discuss the expectations with the stakeholders.

Appendix F
Writing Behavioral Objectives

Behavioral objectives are critical components of any instructional design, including healthcare simulation. They clearly define what learners should be able to do as a result of the training. Behavioral objectives guide the design, development, and evaluation of the simulation, ensuring alignment between the instructional goals and learner outcomes. This appendix provides a comprehensive guide to writing effective behavioral objectives.

What Are Behavioral Objectives?

Behavioral objectives describe the observable and measurable behaviors that learners should demonstrate after completing the training. They focus on what the learner will do, not what the instructor will teach. This learner-centered approach ensures clarity and accountability in educational outcomes.

Key Components of Behavioral Objectives

An effective behavioral objective includes three essential components, often referred to as the **ABC model**:

- **Audience (A)**
    - Specifies who the objective is for (e.g., learners, participants, nursing staff).
    - *Example:* "The nursing student will..."

- **Behavior (B)**
    - Describes the specific, observable action the learner will perform.
    - Use action verbs from **Bloom's Taxonomy**, such as:
    - Cognitive domain (knowledge): *define, explain, analyze*.
    - Psychomotor domain (skills): *perform, demonstrate, administer*.
    - Affective domain (attitudes): *value, advocate, respect*.
    - *Example:* "...perform chest compressions..."

- **Condition (C)**
  - Outlines the conditions under which the behavior will occur. This may include tools, resources, or specific scenarios.
  - *Example:* "…using a high-fidelity mannequin in a simulated cardiac arrest scenario…"

- **Degree (D)**
  - Specifies the criteria for acceptable performance, such as accuracy, time, or quality.
  - Example: "…at a compression depth of 5–6 cm and a rate of 100–120 per minute."

Steps to Write Behavioral Objectives

1. **Start with the End in Mind**
   - Ask yourself: What should learners be able to do after the simulation?
   - *Example:* Manage a patient in septic shock.

2. **Choose an Action Verb**
   - Use verbs that clearly describe observable behaviors.
   - Avoid vague terms like *understand* or *know*, as they are difficult to measure.

3. **Define the Context**
   - Identify the conditions or tools learners will use.

   Example: During a simulated trauma scenario, learners will use standard resuscitation equipment.

4. **Set the Performance Standard**
   - Determine the criteria for success.

   Example: The learner will administer the correct dose of medication within two minutes.

5. **Combine All Elements**

- Combine the audience, behavior, condition, and degree into a single, concise statement.
- *Example:* "The nursing student will administer epinephrine intramuscularly within 30 seconds of recognizing anaphylaxis during a simulated emergency scenario."

Examples of Behavioral Objectives

Cognitive Domain (Knowledge)
- "The medical student will identify the early signs of sepsis based on provided patient charts within five minutes."
- "The participant will explain the sequence of actions in the ACLS algorithm during a debriefing session."

Psychomotor Domain (Skills)
- "The paramedic will perform bag-mask ventilation on a pediatric mannequin for one minute without leaks."
- "The learner will insert an IV catheter in a simulated patient with 90% accuracy on the first attempt."

Affective Domain (Attitudes)
- "The participant will demonstrate empathy by maintaining eye contact and using active listening techniques during a patient interview."
- "The nurse will advocate for patient safety by speaking up during a simulated team handoff when an error is identified."

Tips for Writing Effective Behavioral Objectives
- **Be Specific and Clear**
    - Avoid vague or overly broad statements. Objectives should describe a single behavior.
- **Make Them Measurable**
    - Ensure that the behavior can be observed and assessed.
- **Focus on the Learner**
    - Frame objectives around what the learner will do, not the instructor.
- **Match Objectives to Training Goals**

- o   Align behavioral objectives with the broader goals of the simulation or program.
- **Incorporate Realistic Conditions**
  Use conditions that reflect the clinical environment to increase relevance.

Common Mistakes to Avoid

- **Using Non-Actionable Verbs**
  - o   Avoid terms like *know*, *understand*, or *appreciate* that are subjective and not directly measurable.

- **Being Too General**
  - o   Objectives like "improve communication skills" are too vague. Instead, specify the type of communication and the criteria for success.

- **Failing to Include Performance Criteria**
  - o   Objectives without standards for performance can lead to inconsistent evaluation.

- **Ignoring the Learning Domain**
  - o   Ensure that objectives address the appropriate domain (cognitive, psychomotor, affective) based on the training focus.

Writing clear and measurable behavioral objectives is foundational in developing effective healthcare simulation programs. These objectives not only guide the design and delivery of the training but also ensure alignment between instructional goals and learner outcomes. By following the principles outlined in this appendix, educators and instructional designers can create specific, actionable, and impactful objectives, driving meaningful improvements in learner performance and patient care.

Appendix G
Templates

SAMPLE Scenario Planning Template

Field	Example
Scenario Title	Managing Sepsis in the Emergency Department
Author(s)	Smuckatelli, MD
Dates of Development	2/2025
Department/Organization	Emergency Department
Learning Objectives	1. Recognize early signs of sepsis. 2. Initiate appropriate treatment within 30 minutes. 3. Communicate effectively with team members.
Target Audience	Emergency department nurses and junior physicians.
Crosswalk to applicable Standards (ACGME, CCNE, AACN, etc…)	1. Patient Care 2. Medical Knowledge 3. Interpersonal and Communication Skills
Clinical Context	Emergency department setting with a high-acuity patient presenting with fever and hypotension.
Key Events and Triggers	- Patient presents with tachycardia and low blood pressure. - Sudden oxygen desaturation requiring intervention. - Lab results confirming elevated lactate levels.
General Flow	Patient will present in a bed. Providers will interview the patient and request lab work. The simulation lab will provide the providers lab results. The providers will sselect an appropriate treatment.

Patient Details	68-year-old male with a history of diabetes presenting with fever, confusion, and low urine output.
Learner Roles	- Primary nurse responsible for monitoring vitals and administering fluids. - Physician responsible for ordering tests and initiating antibiotics. - Respiratory therapist providing oxygen support.
Equipment Needs and Resources	- High-fidelity mannequin. - Simulated patient monitor displaying vitals. - IV fluids and medications. - Lab result cards for lactate and blood cultures.
Estimated Time Allocation	- Pre-simulation briefing: 10 minutes. - Simulation scenario: 20 minutes. - Debriefing: 30 minutes.
Desired Outcomes	- Learners recognize sepsis early and initiate a sepsis protocol. - Effective team communication and role delegation. - Timely administration of fluids and antibiotics.
Facilitator Notes	- Introduce subtle early signs of sepsis to assess recognition skills. - Escalate patient deterioration if treatment is delayed.
Debriefing Points	- Importance of early recognition and intervention. - Reflection on team communication and role clarity. - Review of sepsis protocol adherence.
Evaluation Criteria	- Timely recognition of sepsis (within 5 minutes). - Proper use of closed-loop communication. - Completion of treatment steps within the allocated time.

Assessment Design Template

Field	Example
Learning Objective	Learners will demonstrate effective team communication during a simulated cardiac arrest.
Assessment Method	Observation and scoring using a structured rubric.
Assessment Tool	Team Communication Rubric (focuses on closed-loop communication, leadership, and clarity).
Performance Criteria	1. Verbalizes clear instructions to the team. 2. Confirms understanding using closed-loop communication. 3. Maintains role clarity under pressure.
Performance Level	- *Excellent:* All criteria consistently met throughout the simulation. - *Satisfactory:* Most criteria met, with occasional lapses. - *Needs Improvement:* Significant lapses in communication or clarity.
Weighting (if applicable)	30% of the overall simulation performance score.
Evaluator Role	Facilitator observes and scores using the rubric.
Feedback Plan	Feedback provided during the debriefing session, focusing on strengths and areas for improvement.
Alignment with Learning Objectives	The assessment aligns with the learning objective by evaluating the ability to demonstrate clear and effective team communication.
Notes/Comments	Observers should focus on key moments, such as role delegation and responses to critical events.

Resource Planning Template

Field	Example
Resource Category	Equipment
Specific Resource	High-fidelity Manikin
Quantity Needed	1
Estimated Cost	See fee structure
Source/Provider	Laerdal SimMan
Preparation Requirements	Calibrate vitals monitor, preload scenario, and perform function check
Responsible Person	Jane Doe (simulation specialist)
Notes/Comments	None

Field	Example
Resource Category	Personnel
Specific Resource	Facilitator with EM expertise
Quantity Needed	1
Estimated Cost	N/A
Source/Provider	In-house faculty
Preparation Requirements	Review facilitator guide, scenario, and attend pre-brief
Responsible Person	John Smith (Sim Coordinator)
Notes/Comments	None

Pilot Testing Template

Field	Example
Simulation Title	Managing Sepsis in the Emergency Department
Pilot Test Date	September 20, 2023
Participants	3 Emergency Department nurses, 1 junior physician
Facilitator	Jane Doe (Simulation Coordinator)
Key Objectives Tested	1. Recognizing early signs of sepsis. 2. Initiating the sepsis protocol. 3. Effective team communication.
Strength of Simulation	Realistic patient deterioration events were effective for triggering learner

DESIGN, DEVELOP, DELIVER: USING ADDIE TO BUILD EFFECTIVE HEALTHCARE SIMULATIONS

	actions. Scenario setup and environment felt authentic.
Areas for Improvement	Instructions for the initial task (ordering blood cultures) were unclear to participants. Timing of critical events felt too rushed.
Clarity of Instructions	Participants noted that some steps in the patient history collection required clarification.
Realism of Scenario	Scenario felt highly realistic, but one participant suggested adding more background details about the patient's history.
Effectiveness of Equipment/Resources	Monitors and vital sign readouts were accurate and easy to use, but the IV pump was difficult to operate.
Feedback on Timing and Flow	Patient deterioration escalated too quickly, leaving participants feeling overwhelmed. Suggested extending the timeline by 5 minutes.
Additional Comments	Include a brief pre-simulation briefing on recognizing sepsis criteria. Update facilitator guide with clearer instructions for the opening task.

Learner Orientation Checklist

☐	Receive and review pre-simulation materials (e.g., objectives, case studies, protocols).
☐	Understand the purpose and goals of the simulation session.
☐	Familiarize with the simulation environment (e.g., equipment, layout).
☐	Introduce key personnel, including facilitators and observers.
☐	Explain roles and expectations for all participants.
☐	Discuss confidentiality agreements and psychological safety rules.
☐	Provide a walkthrough of the simulation process (briefing, simulation, debriefing).
☐	Ensure learners understand the evaluation criteria and methods.

☐	Confirm readiness to engage in the simulation (e.g., mental preparation, comfort).
☐	Address questions or concerns from participants before starting.

Appendix H
Sample Simulation Events Table

State	Patient Status	Student Actions & Triggers	
1. Baseline		Desired Actions:	Instructions for Operator: • Triggers: •
2.		Desired Actions:	Instructions for Operator: • Triggers: •
3.		Desired Actions:	Instructions for Operator: • Triggers: •
4.		Desired Actions:	Instructions for Operator: • Triggers: •

This table is very common in simulation scenario templates.

Program should adapt the table to meet their educational needs.

Additional columns used can include:
- Patient Dialogue
- Patient History
- Branching for desired and undesired events
- State timeframe

Appendix I
Best Practices for Using Focus Groups During the Analysis Phase

Focus groups are a valuable tool during the Analysis phase of the ADDIE model. They offer qualitative insights into learner needs, gaps in performance, and organizational objectives. By facilitating guided discussions among stakeholders, focus groups provide rich, context-specific data that can inform the design and development of effective training programs. However, focus groups must be carefully planned, facilitated, and analyzed to maximize effectiveness.

Why Use Focus Groups in the Analysis Phase?
Focus groups allow instructional designers to:
- Gather diverse perspectives from key stakeholders, including learners, facilitators, and subject matter experts (SMEs).
- Identify specific performance gaps and challenges in the workplace or clinical environment.
- Explore underlying factors contributing to these gaps, such as communication issues, resource limitations, or workflow inefficiencies.
- Generate ideas for potential training solutions that are practical and relevant to the target audience.

Focus groups can uncover nuanced needs that surveys or performance reports might overlook by engaging participants in collaborative discussions.

Best Practices for Conducting Focus Groups

1. Define the Purpose
Before conducting a focus group, clearly articulate its purpose and objectives. This ensures that the discussion remains focused and aligns with the goals of the Analysis phase.

Example: For a healthcare simulation on sepsis management, the focus group's purpose might be to explore gaps in recognizing and responding to early signs of sepsis.

2. Select the Right Participants

Choose a diverse group of participants who can provide meaningful input. Ensure that stakeholders represent various perspectives, such as:

- **Learners**: Those who will participate in the training.
- **Facilitators**: Educators or trainers who deliver the content.
- **SMEs**: Clinicians or professionals with expertise in the subject matter.
- **Administrators**: Decision-makers who understand organizational goals and constraints.

Tip: Keep the group size between 6 and 12 participants to ensure active engagement and manageable discussion dynamics.

3. Develop a Structured Discussion Guide

Prepare a discussion guide with open-ended questions that align with the focus group's purpose. Organize questions into key themes, such as:

- **Current Practices:** "What challenges do you face when managing sepsis cases?"
- **Learning Needs:** "What skills or knowledge gaps do you think need to be addressed?"
- **Barriers to Success:** "What factors prevent optimal performance in this area?"
- **Desired Outcomes:** "What would an ideal training program look like for this topic?"

4. Create a Comfortable Environment

Set the stage for open and honest discussions by creating a safe and comfortable environment:

- Choose a neutral location, whether in person or virtual, that minimizes power dynamics or intimidation.
- Establish ground rules, such as mutual respect, confidentiality, and active listening.
- Begin with icebreakers or simple introductory questions to ease participants into the discussion.

5. Facilitate, Do not Dominate
The facilitator's role is to guide the conversation, not control it. Encourage active participation from all members while keeping the discussion on track.

- **Techniques for Effective Facilitation:**
    - Use probing questions: "Can you elaborate on that point?"
    - Redirect dominant participants: "Thank you. Let's hear from someone else on this topic."
    - Address silence: "Does anyone have a different perspective?"

6. Record and Document the Discussion
Record the session (with participants' consent) and assign a note-taker to document key points to ensure accurate data collection. Tools such as transcription software can streamline the process for virtual focus groups.

- **Key Data to Capture:**
    - Recurring themes and ideas.
    - Specific challenges and suggestions.
    - Nonverbal cues, such as enthusiasm or hesitation, indicate participant priorities.

7. Analyze the Data
After the focus group, review the recordings, notes, and transcripts to identify key findings. Use thematic analysis to group similar responses and uncover patterns.

- **Steps for Analysis:**
    - Highlight recurring themes, such as communication challenges or resource constraints.
    - Identify unique insights or suggestions that may inform the training program.
    - Compare focus group data with other analysis methods (e.g., surveys or performance metrics) to triangulate findings.

8. Use Focus Group Insights Effectively

Translate focus group findings into actionable inputs for the Design phase:

- Develop training objectives based on identified gaps.
- Tailor scenarios to address real-world challenges described by participants.
- Incorporate suggestions from learners and SMEs to enhance relevance and engagement.

Example Focus Group in Practice

Scenario: A hospital identifies frequent delays in administering antibiotics for septic patients.

Focus Group Purpose: Explore barriers to timely intervention and gather input for a simulation-based training program.

Participants: Emergency department nurses, physicians, and pharmacists.

Key Findings:

- Nurses report delays due to unclear protocols during shift changes.
- Physicians express difficulty in identifying early signs of sepsis among patients with complex conditions.
- Pharmacists suggest streamlining the antibiotic request process to reduce bottlenecks.

Outcome:

Based on the focus group data, the training program emphasizes communication during handoffs, early recognition of sepsis, and collaboration with pharmacy services.

Benefits of Focus Groups in the Analysis Phase

- **Rich Qualitative Data:** Focus groups provide context and depth that quantitative methods alone cannot capture.
- **Stakeholder Buy-In:** Engaging stakeholders fosters a sense of ownership and increases support for the training program.
- **Targeted Solutions:** Insights from focus groups ensure that the training addresses real-world challenges and learner needs.

Conclusion

Focus groups are a powerful tool for gathering qualitative data during the Analysis phase of ADDIE. By following best practices—such as selecting diverse participants, using a structured discussion guide, and analyzing data effectively—focus groups can uncover valuable insights that shape meaningful and impactful training programs. In healthcare simulation, these insights ensure that training solutions are not only relevant but also aligned with the complex realities of clinical practice.

Appendix J
Learning Theories

Aspect	Behaviorism	Cognitivism	Constructivism	Connectionism
Focus	Observable behavior and responses to stimuli	Internal mental processes like memory and problem-solving	Learner's construction of knowledge through experience	Connections between concepts, skills, and behaviors
Key Theorists	B.F. Skinner, Ivan Pavlov, John Watson	Jean Piaget, Jerome Bruner, Robert Gagné	Lev Vygotsky, John Dewey, Jean Piaget	Edward Thorndike, David Ausubel
Mechanism of Learning	Conditioning through reinforcement and punishment	Information processing, schema development, and organization	Active engagement, exploration, and reflection	Creating associations between stimuli, responses, and outcomes
Role of the Learner	Passive recipient of stimuli	Active processor of information	Active participant in creating meaning	Active network-builder connecting ideas
Role of the Instructor	Deliverer of reinforcement or punishment	Facilitator of knowledge organization	Guide or mentor supporting discovery	Designer of environments promoting strong connections
Application	Repetition, rewards, and punishments for skill acquisition	Use of scaffolding, concept mapping, and structured guidance	Collaborative activities, hands-on exploration	Linking prior knowledge to new concepts
Strengths	Effective for developing	Enhances problem-	Encourages creativity,	Supports personalized

Aspect	Behaviorism	Cognitivism	Constructivism	Connectionism
	basic skills and habits	solving and higher-order thinking	autonomy, and critical thinking	learning and integration of ideas
Limitations	Ignores mental processes and intrinsic motivation	May overlook individual differences and social context	Can lack structure and be time-intensive	Limited empirical research and overemphasis on connections

Summary of Learning Theories

1. Behaviorism

Behaviorism focuses on observable behavior, emphasizing the role of environmental stimuli in shaping learner responses. Through reinforcement and punishment, learners acquire specific skills or behaviors. This theory works well for foundational learning tasks, such as memorization or motor skills. However, its lack of attention to mental processes and intrinsic motivation can limit its application to complex or abstract learning scenarios.

2. Cognitivism

Cognitivism shifts the focus from external behaviors to internal mental processes. Learning is seen as acquiring and organizing knowledge through schema development and problem-solving. C scaffolding, concept mapping, and structured guidance help learners connect new information with existing knowledge. While highly effective for teaching critical thinking and problem-solving, it may overlook the social and emotional contexts of learning.

3. Constructivism

Constructivism posits that learners actively construct knowledge through hands-on experiences and reflection. It emphasizes collaboration, creativity, and real-world application. Constructivist approaches are especially valuable for fostering deeper understanding and learner autonomy. However, this theory's unstructured nature may make it time-intensive and less suitable for environments that require rapid skill acquisition.

4. Connectionism

Connectionism focuses on building associations between ideas, skills, and behaviors. Learning is viewed as forming a network of interconnected concepts, with new knowledge linked to prior experiences. This theory supports personalized and contextualized learning environments. While promising, connectionism's application is still emerging, and it may overemphasize connections without sufficient empirical support.

Each theory offers unique insights into learning and serves different educational contexts. Behaviorism is ideal for skill-based tasks, cognitivism supports structured problem-solving, constructivism fosters exploration and creativity, and connectionism emphasizes personalized learning. In practice, a blended approach often yields the best results, leveraging the strengths of each theory to address diverse learner needs and instructional goals.

Appendix K
Glossary

This glossary provides definitions of key terms used throughout the chapters, offering clarity and context for their application in the ADDIE model and healthcare simulation.

3D Model of Debriefing
A debriefing framework that includes three stages: Defuse (process emotions), Discover (analyze actions), and Deepen (connect to broader concepts). Often used in simulation-based learning to guide reflection.

ADDIE Model
A systematic instructional design framework comprising five phases: Analyze, Design, Develop, Implement, and Evaluate. Widely used in educational and training programs, including healthcare simulation.

Adult Learning Principles
Theories focusing on how adults learn, emphasizing practical application, self-direction, and leveraging prior experience. Key to designing healthcare simulations.

Behavioral Objectives
Specific, measurable statements that describe what learners will be able to do as a result of training. Often structured using the ABCD model (Audience, Behavior, Condition, Degree).

Bloom's Taxonomy
A framework for categorizing educational goals, focusing on six levels of cognitive learning: Remember, Understand, Apply, Analyze, Evaluate, and Create.

Checklist
An evaluation tool that outlines specific steps or criteria to be performed during a task. Used to ensure consistency and thoroughness in assessments.

Cognitivism
A learning theory focusing on internal mental processes, such as memory and problem-solving, emphasizing the importance of schema and scaffolding in learning.

Connectionism
A theory of learning emphasizing the creation of associations between ideas, skills, or behaviors. Learning occurs through the formation and strengthening of these connections.

Constructivism
A learning theory suggesting that learners actively construct knowledge through experiences and reflection, emphasizing collaboration and real-world application.

Continuous Improvement
An iterative process of refining instructional materials and methods based on feedback and evaluation to enhance outcomes.

Debriefing
A structured discussion following a simulation to reflect on performance, identify strengths and weaknesses, and apply lessons to future scenarios.

Evaluation
The phase in ADDIE where the effectiveness of instructional materials and training programs is assessed. Includes formative and summative evaluations.

Facilitator
An individual responsible for guiding learners through a simulation or training session, ensuring engagement and supporting reflection.

Formative Assessment
Ongoing evaluation is conducted during the learning process to provide immediate feedback for improvement.

High-Fidelity Simulation

A simulation that replicates real-world clinical environments and scenarios with high levels of accuracy and realism.

Iterative Design
An approach to development where materials are continuously refined through cycles of feedback, testing, and improvement.

Learning Objectives
Statements describing the intended outcomes of instruction, specifying what learners will know, do, or feel after training.

Needs Analysis
The process of identifying gaps in knowledge, skills, or performance to inform the development of training programs.

Psychomotor Objectives
Goals that focus on the development of physical skills or tasks, often involving precise movements or manual dexterity.

Reliability
The consistency of an evaluation tool in measuring performance across different evaluators, scenarios, or time periods.

Rubric
A scoring guide used to evaluate learner performance against defined criteria. Includes specific levels of achievement for each criterion.

Scenario Design
The process of creating realistic, evidence-based situations for learners to engage in during a simulation. Scenarios align with learning objectives.

Scaffolding
A teaching technique where support is gradually reduced as learners gain competence, helping them achieve higher levels of understanding.

SMEs (Subject Matter Experts)

Individuals with expertise in a specific domain who contribute to the development and accuracy of instructional materials.

Summative Assessment
Evaluation conducted at the end of a training program to determine if learning objectives were achieved.

Validity
The extent to which an evaluation tool accurately measures what it is intended to measure.

Virtual Reality (VR)
A technology that creates immersive, computer-generated environments for training, enabling learners to practice skills in simulated settings.

About the Author

Keith A. Beaulieu, MBA, BS, BA, CHSOS-A

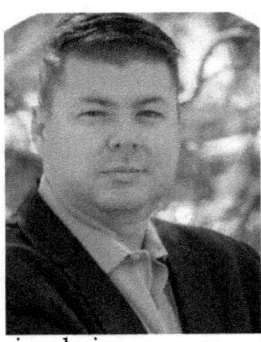

Keith A. Beaulieu is an accomplished professional with extensive experience in healthcare simulation, accreditation management, and operational leadership. Currently serving as the Accreditation and Operations Manager at the Sue & Bill Gross School of Nursing, University of California, Irvine, Keith oversees accreditation processes and ensures operational excellence within the simulation programs.

With a career spanning over a decade in healthcare simulation, Keith has held pivotal roles, including Director of Operations for the Medical Education Simulation Center and Simulation Curriculum Coordinator at prominent institutions. His contributions have directly supported program growth, quality improvement, and alignment with accreditation standards. At the Sue & Bill Gross School of Nursing, Keith has ensured continued program accreditation and approval from the Commission on Collegiate Nursing Education (CCNE) and the California Board of Registered Nursing.

Keith is a Certified Healthcare Simulation Operations Specialist – Advanced (CHSOS-A) and a respected member of the Society for Simulation in Healthcare (SSH) Accreditation Council. He has performed over 30 accreditation site reviews globally for SSH, applying his expertise to enhance simulation programs across diverse healthcare settings. In addition to his site review experience, he has been instrumental in supporting accreditation research and standards development, contributing to the field's growth and innovation.

Keith is also a published author, contributing to **Achieving and Maintaining Accreditation for Nursing School Programs: A Comprehensive Guide** and **Achieving Program Accreditation for Healthcare Simulation Programs: A Resource Guide** and **Simulation Operations in Healthcare Education**, and writing a chapter in the most recent edition of **Defining Excellence in Simulation Programs**. These works reflect his deep knowledge and thought leadership in accreditation and healthcare simulation.

Keith's educational background includes an MBA and multiple leadership, quality improvement, and simulation education certifications. Through his strategic vision, extensive accreditation experience, and scholarly contributions, Keith has become a leading figure in advancing the quality and impact of healthcare simulation worldwide.

Other Titles Available by this Author

Achieving and Maintaining Accreditation for Nursing School Programs:
A Comprehensive Guide

Achieving Program Accreditation for Healthcare Simulation Programs
A Resources Guide

Simulation Operations in Healthcare Education
A Primer into the Role of Operations in Medical and Nursing Programs

HISTORY SERIES

Camp Haan
The History of Riverside's World War II Antiaircraft Training Center

Available on

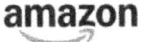

www.ingramcontent.com/pod-product-compliance
Lightning Source LLC
Chambersburg PA
CBHW072150070526
44585CB00015B/1074